Safe Haven

Ellis Amdur, M.A., N.C.C., C.M.H.S.

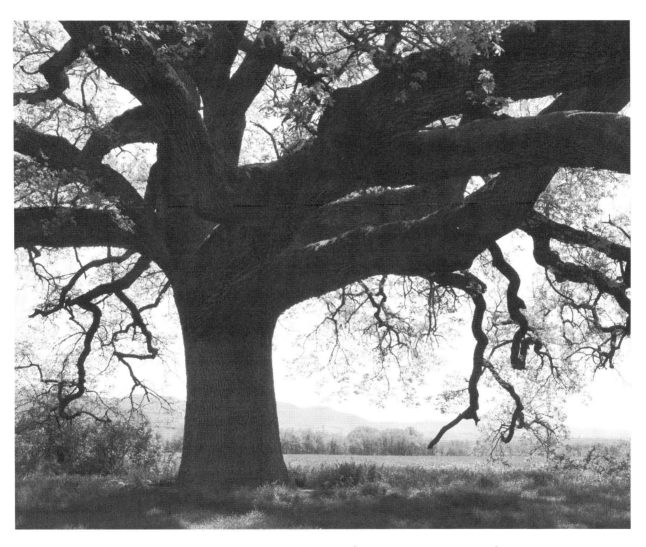

Skills to Calm and De-escalate Aggressive and
Mentally Ill Individuals: 2nd Edition

A Comprehensive Guidebook for

Personnel Working in Hospital

and Residential Settings

An Edgework Book
www.edgework.info

Notes and Notices

Credits

Photographs by: Dreamstime.com
Illustrations by: Shoko Zama
Design: Soundview Design Studio

Contents

In Gratitude for Expert Critique

The following professionals have closely reviewed this book. With each draft, I corrected errors of fact, added new information, and fine-tuned the manuscript. All responsibility for this book, however, must lie in my hands. Any errors, in particular, are my responsibility. Given that people's health, well-being, and on occasion, even their lives can be on the line in work such as you do, please do not hesitate to contact me if you believe that any part of this book is inaccurate or requires additional material. I will revise this book, as needed, in future editions.

Marlene Sassali Burrows, MS, Community Mental Health, Licensed Mental Health Counselor. Ms. Sassali Burrows has over thirty years' experience in community mental health, with twenty-two years working in the area of crisis services. This includes nine years as a Designated Mental Health Professional (responsible for the evaluation of people possibly in need of involuntary psychiatric hospitalization), and thirteen years as a hospital emergency room psychiatric clinician. She is currently the Program Manager for Clark County Crisis Services, in Vancouver, Washington.

Bea Dixon, PhD, founder of Stand and Live, the original publisher of my work. I worked in close collaboration with Dr. Dixon for a number of years on this and other projects, and simply put, this book would not exist without her work with me.

Cheryl S. Reynolds, MD, is a Fellow of the American College of Emergency Physicians and Certified Professional in Health Care Risk Management.

Paul Schweer, writer, gave invaluable advice on style and format.

Mark Sexton is a lead instructor of Prevention and Management of Assaultive Behavior (PMAB) for the Providence Hospital systems in Portland, Oregon, and part of the team responsible for re-authorship of Providence Hospital's training program on the same subject.

Introduction

This book is designed to address the unique challenges facing personnel working in inpatient and residential settings when dealing with mentally ill and aggressive patients. This includes those in mental health services, inpatient drug/alcohol treatment facilities, and such professionals as psychologists, therapists, psychiatrists, counselors, case managers, security staff and social workers, as well as nurses and doctors working in hospitals or nursing homes. Although some information is focused on interventions specific to patients who have a diagnosis of mental illness, many strategies also apply to patients who are admitted to general and specialty units, such as internal medicine, neurology, ICU, CCU, post-op units, and the like.

We do not have the luxury of diagnosis in potentially dangerous situations. Rather, the patient must be stabilized so that diagnosis is possible. For this reason, the focus of this book is on behavior, not specific diagnosis. Anyone manifesting extreme emotional disturbance, or behaviors affected by distortions of perception and cognition, will be regarded in this text as "mentally ill," whether the cause is a genuine mental disorder, intoxication, a disease process, or a momentary aberration due to stress, grief, or frustration. There is no doubt that *clinical* treatment of any of these individuals may be markedly different: de-escalation of aggression, however, focuses on the behavior of the person, not the cause. On the other hand, there is absolutely nothing here that conflicts with clinical treatment, and those for whom this is a direct responsibility will find that this approach to people will provide access routes toward clinically appropriate communication.

The behaviors of mentally ill individuals can be quite bizarre and hard to understand. What we cannot understand is unpredictable, and therefore seems to be dangerous, even when it is not. By learning the meaning of their behaviors, such people become more comprehensible. Through such understanding, you will become more skillful in assessing if a person – mentally ill, drug intoxicated, or simply very distressed – is truly dangerous. In many situations, you will have the ability to calm them as well.

The ability to recognize and de-escalate dangerous and manipulative behaviors will make you far better at your job. You will begin to demonstrate "grace under fire," the ability to become the center of gravity within a situation so that it coalesces into an ordered system around you. You will display a kind of power that draws people to you rather than makes them bend in submission.

It is my hope that this volume, which encompasses over 25 years of experience in face-to-face encounters with mentally ill and emotionally disturbed individuals, will be invaluable in readying you for such encounters.

This book is one of a series of books I have written for people who must face aggressive individuals. Other books in these series are specific to those who work in social services agencies, as 9-1-1 dispatchers, police officers, probation/parole officers, corporate security officers, fire fighters, corrections officers, and emergency medical technicians.

I have also written a separate version for people who live with mentally ill family members. It is not enough that hospital personnel have the skills to calm patients on the relatively infrequent occasions that you see them. Those who live with them on a daily basis – their family – need these skills even more. A culture of safety should encompass the entirety of your patients' lives. In so doing, there will be fewer occasions when de-escalation techniques, much less hospitalization, are even necessary. I strongly encourage you to ensure that the families of your patients are made aware of, or if possible, are provided with these books, so that they, too, can take part in an overarching ethos of protection for themselves, for you, and for those people whose care and safety we have all taken responsibility.

Please refer to my website www.edgework.info for more information.

A Note on Terminology

The word hospital has the same roots as the words hostel and hotel, and it originally referred to a place for the reception and lodging of pilgrims and strangers. The word has permutated to refer, variously, to a place of lodging for the indigent, the destitute, the infirm, and the young.

According to the Oxford English Dictionary, the modern usage refers to "an institution or establishment for the care of the sick or wounded, or for those who required medical treatment."

It will be quite unwieldy for me to refer to all of the various types of inpatient institutions by name in each sentence of the text, among them being ordinary hospitals, inpatient mental health institutions, drug and alcohol residential treatment facilities, and residential care facilities, to name only a few. Therefore, aside from such general terms as "institution," I will use the word "hospital" in the broadest sense, meaning any facility that lodges and/or treats the sick, the wounded, the destitute, or those requiring care on an ongoing basis.

Preface

What is a mental illness anyway? Is it any odd or eccentric behavior, or should we confine the term for more serious disturbances of behavior and thought? It sometimes seems that we lump together mental phenomenon as disparate as the distinction between a common cold and lung cancer. Yes, both may make breathing difficult, but they are very different disorders.

Not everyone who needs to be calmed or de-escalated is aggressive. Those who display unusual or eccentric patterns of behavior are more difficult to communicate with, and when people's ability to communicate breaks down, the risk of aggression increases.

Beyond aggression, however, people who display such patterns of behavior have a more difficult time getting help, both in expressing their needs and taking in information when it is offered. This can be frustrating for both of you. When you can recognize the pattern of communication that such people display, as well as understand how best to "get through" to them, you have a greater opportunity to respond to them in an ethical and caring manner.

The initial sections of this book (Sections I – III) offer detailed descriptions of the most significant behaviors that mentally ill patients may display, regardless of diagnosis. Along with each description of behavior are suggestions for the best way to communicate with such a person. It is unavoidable that when you read something in sequence it will seem that the advice given for a syndrome or behavior is THE procedure to do. However, all of the strategies described here overlap. Some are applicable with almost any type of individual, while others are specific to only one type of behavior or symptom. People are very complex – and this, of course, includes people who have a mental illness. Just because you might be reading about delusions or hallucinations, for example, doesn't mean that the patient is not also disorganized, intoxicated, or manic. What you are trying to develop through this book is a "skill map": a range of communication tactics that cover many situations.

The establishment of safety and the de-escalation of aggression are the primary purposes of this book, so the focus here will be on general patterns of communication and behavior, *regardless* of the cause. Mental illness, in this vein, does not just refer to such disorders as schizophrenia, bipolar disorder, or depression. For example, intoxication can be considered a time-limited, substance-induced mental disorder. For a number of reasons, some people, otherwise normal, can display acute, "out of character" behaviors, due to problems or stressors in their lives. Thus, for the sake of this discussion, substance abuse, neurological disorders, and atypical episodes brought on by stress or other factors all can manifest as mental illness.

The cause may be relevant if making appropriate referrals for treatment: in crisis, however, we should most emphatically focus on the behaviors, whatever the cause.

Section IV is the heart of the book; it focuses on the one aspect of de-escalation that we have the opportunity to exert total control: ourselves. This section offers strategies to hone your intuition so that you become aware of other people's distress or potential danger as early as possible. It also offers strategies to calm and center yourself so that, rather than contribute to a crisis, your presence calms and gives strength.

The middle sections of the book (Sections V – IX) specifically address crisis situations that present risk to both the patient and to other people: suicide and inter-personal aggression. You will learn to recognize patterns of behavior that enable you to identify modes of aggression, be it self-destructive behavior or potential violence toward others, as well as best-practice interventions to de-escalate people manifesting these different types of aggression, whatever their diagnosis may be.

Section X focuses on the creation of a "culture of safety," what is necessary to establish a safe environment within your hospital.

Perhaps your worst fear is that you will get hurt or even killed by an aggressor. This guidebook will NOT teach you methods of physical self-defense. If you genuinely need training in force-on-force self-defense, which includes evasion, breaking free of holds, or in the worst cases, fighting back against an attacker, your local police department, hospital, or sexual assault crisis center may have references to reputable groups. I will also not teach you how to put a person in restraints. Those tactics need to be learned firsthand and cannot be addressed in a text.

The Undamaged Self

You are walking outside on an icy winter day. You slip suddenly and spin toward the pavement. At the last minute, you thrust out an arm that breaks your fall. It also breaks your right wrist. Your life, for a few weeks or months, is different. Suddenly, even the simplest daily tasks are difficult and may require assistance. Still, even though you are inconvenienced, and the injury probably changes your mood quite a bit, you are still "you," the same person as before your injury. In due time, your injuries will heal, the accident will be forgotten, and you will continue through life. However, such is not the case with mental illness.

Severe mental illness can cause mental and emotional disturbances far more profound than the temporary inconveniences brought on by physical injury. One's ability to think is distorted, and delusions skew reality. Perceptions may be bizarre, even hallucinatory. Emotions swing from high to low, or shift into realms at odds with one's immediate circumstances. Mental illness is an assault on one's worldview.

Yet, there is still a person behind the symptoms. The patient under your care is not simply a bundle of raw emotions or distorted cognitions. The philosophy of this book can be summed up in a single phrase: you can choose to speak to the illness, or speak to the *person* who is ill. Of course, mere words do not cure severe mental illness. Nonetheless, there exists an essential part of them untouched by their mental illness. That core part of their psyche, the *undamaged self,* is the person you are trying to reach.

SECTION I

Working with Those with
Unusual, Intense, or Eccentric
Communication Styles

CHAPTER 1

Tell It Like It Is: Communication
with Concrete Thinkers

Concrete thinkers have a lot of difficulty, or even a complete inability, to understand metaphors, slang, or imagery. Instead, they take everything you say literally. For example:

- "Way to go!" an expression meant as praise. The concrete individual thinks, "I'm not going anywhere," or "Where?" or "Do they want me to leave now?"
- "Don't give me any attitude," an expression that means that the person shouldn't be oppositional or aggressive. The concrete individual thinks, "I'm not giving them anything," or "My attitudes are mine. How do I give them?"
- "OK. So you don't have to worry any more. The nurse will be here shortly. I want you to hold the cloth on your arm and press it really firmly, so that you don't bleed. Just look in my eyes. Listen to what I'm saying. The nurse will be here in just a minute."

Consider this last example. It is far more effective to "break" your communication up into single items. Your tone of voice should be firm, calm, reassuring. Repeat phrases when they have not registered it the first time. <u>Shouting to "get through" to the person will only make things worse.</u>

Example: Communication with someone displaying concrete thinking
- The nurse is coming.
- Hold the cloth hard on your arm.
- Yes, really hard.
- I know you are bleeding. I'm holding the cloth on your leg, and you hold the one on your arm.
- Good. Hold the cloth on your arm.
- Hold the cloth on your arm.
- Hold the cloth on your arm.
- I know it's scary. The nurse will be here in a little while. She's going to help you.

Review: Concrete Thinkers

You will recognize concrete thinkers because they take what you say literally. Therefore be sure to:

- Use clear, short sentences, with a firm, calm voice.
- Give directions using simple words that are easy to understand.
- Show a minimum of emotion. Don't get irritated when they don't immediately understand you. They respond much more to your tone of voice than to what you say.

CHAPTER 2

Rigid Personality (Asperger's Syndrome, "High Functioning Autism," and Other Similar Disorders)

Individuals with a "rigid personality" are often very intelligent, socially withdrawn people who may live their lives mostly in an online environment. They frequently display the full range of behaviors that merit the diagnosis of Asperger's syndrome. They may have tremendous difficulty negotiating social interactions. They find other people to be incomprehensible, confusing, or threatening. They can have tremendous difficulty understanding what others are thinking or feeling from their facial expressions, body posture, and vocal tone. Other people, particularly some individuals with schizophrenia, often show a similar combination of "cluelessness" and rigidity in communication with others. Such rigid personalities can become fixated on their own preoccupations and imagine that everyone else shares them.

Example: A child with rigid thinking fixates on one subject

A therapist asks a child with Asperger's syndrome what he thought the bully, who was beating him up, was thinking. "Oh, he was thinking of Lewis and Clark." Astonished, the therapist asks why the bully would be thinking of that. The child replies, "What else could he be thinking about? Lewis and Clark took the greatest journey . . ." It takes a good ten minutes for the therapist to get him off the subject.

They can also be very literal (concrete), and they can get stuck on thoughts and behaviors (obsessive). Others are simply not interested in or aware of other's feelings. This can lead them to be very blunt or painfully honest.

Examples: The painful honesty of the rigid personality
- "What is that on your face. Rosacea, I'm guessing, unless it's some kind of rash. You better hope it is a rash because there's no cure for rosacea and it just gets worse and worse. Many people end up with deformed faces because of it."
- "You've gained a lot of weight in the last year. I don't mind, but many men think that is disgusting."

When attempting to calm a person who displays a rigid personality, stating and reiterating the rules is the first method of intervention. State each rule in a matter-of-fact way, as if simply providing information. Follow this up with a logical sequence of steps to resolve their problem. Attempts at validating their feelings will often merely result in the patient becoming increasingly confused or upset, as will talking about *your* feelings. You must be as concrete and literal as they are.

Try to avoid physical contact. Many such people detest even the lightest touch and can react violently.

Example: De-escalation with a person with a rigid personality

Pavel: "Someone has taken my book! No one is allowed to touch my book or any of my things! Someone is going to get socked right now!"

Staff person: "Pavel, I want to hear about this, but the rule is no yelling in the building. Stop yelling, and tell me about your book!"

Pavel: "But I want to yell. I am very angry."

Staff person: "But you must not yell. It is against the rules here."

Pavel: "I think that is a stupid rule! I am angry and want to yell."

Staff person: "It is still the rule. Stop shouting and we will talk."

Pavel (*in a quiet voice, but clenching his fists and pounding them together*): "I'm really mad about my book. Someone took it."

Staff person: "Pavel, I really want to hear about this, but you must remember that we have another rule. No pounding your fists together."

Pavel: "That is another stupid rule."

(*Eventually, Pavel sits and quietly talks.*)

Staff person: "You are really upset about not knowing where your book is. You are also upset that someone may have borrowed it or touched it. Let's go to your room and look for it."

In some group homes or other community settings (and even individual residences), staff or family set up a designated place to express intolerable emotions. Some people with rigid personalities, who do not want to hurt or hit anyone, still need a way to discharge tension. Without such an option, they feel like they are going to explode. They can go to this safe room and yell for a while, or pound a heavy bag or pillow, and then return to solve the problem. However, please refer to the discussion on venting (Chapter 46). It is only through careful work together and a long-term relationship that you will learn if such strong expressions of emotions are actually calming or stimulating – the latter leading to dangerous escalation.

Review: Communication with rigid personalities

You will recognize the patient with a rigid personality because they get stuck on subjects that seem rather odd in relation to the current circumstances. Furthermore, they seem out-of-sync with society and unconscious of their effect on others. When calming or de-escalating these patients, you should do the following:

- State the rules in a matter-of-fact way, as if providing information.
- Follow up with a logical sequence of steps to solve their problem.
- Caution: validating their feelings will very likely confuse and distress them, as will talking about *your* feelings.

CHAPTER 3

Information Processing and Retention:
Consolidating Gains

Being mentally ill requires considerable survival skills. Imagine trying to stand upright in a windstorm, or trying to have all your conversations in noisy restaurants, no matter how important the subject. One skill that many mentally ill people develop is the art of "faking normal." People around them may do frightening things, but they don't show their fear. Other people may anger them, but they smile and pretend everything is all right. Conversations and ideas may be too complex, too fast, too metaphoric or irrelevant to what is going on inside them, but they have learned to pick up the rhythm of the other person's speech, nod at the right moments, smile or laugh when needed, and agree with the tag lines that invite such agreement. (You may also have seen similar behaviors among people for whom English is not their first language.)

Therefore, *particularly* when in discussion with a mentally ill or emotionally upset patient, never assume that they understand just because they have either said that they do or nodded at the right moment. You need to check to see that you do, in fact, understand one another. There are several ways to do this:

The least effective method is to repeat yourself, using other words, if they have either tuned you out or didn't understand you the first time. They may merely fake understanding again.

The difference between repetition as a de-escalation tactic and as a method of confirming understanding

This is different from the repetition you must do with the latent (Chapter 15) or concrete thinker (Chapter 1), when you DO repeat yourself when giving instructions. In those cases, you are repeating to help the person track what you are saying. However, simply repeating yourself and assuming the other person understands what you've said is often a mistake.

Have the patient repeat back your instructions. This can be very useful, but there are times when this, too, can be problematic, because some people may simply echo what you are saying without any comprehension.

Use open sentences. "So, Diane, if I've got it right, I will call your doctor tomorrow and explain the problem. And you will …" Of course, you hope that she will fill in the rest of the sentence. If not, you have some more explaining to do.

Write down the most important points. Many people do not assimilate a lot of information that they hear, no matter how hard they listen. In these situations, you may find that writing down on a 3 x 5 card the most important points of your conversation or agreement is beneficial to their understanding. You give them the card, review the points, and tell them to check the card if they have difficulty remembering what they are supposed to do.

Review: How to consolidate gains
- The least effective way is to simply repeat yourself, hoping that their replies really mean that they understand.
- Have the patient repeat back your instructions.
- Use open sentences and questions, allowing the patient to fill in the blanks.
- Write down the most important points of understanding on a card as a point of reference.

CHAPTER 4

Coping with Stubborn Refusals

There are many occasions when, despite treating your patient with respect and understanding, they refuse to comply with suggestions or directives, maintaining their defiance even in the face of possible sanctions. For example, a patient won't take her medications, bathe, respect the right of others to speak in group sessions, fill out paperwork, or comply with treatment recommendations.

If you have been bossing your patient around, patronizing them, or treating them with disrespect, it would not be surprising if they resist you.
All people – mentally ill or not – have pride, and no one likes another person talking down to them or controlling their lives.

Authoritarian behavior is also very dangerous. It is surely a high risk factor in assaults on staff by mentally ill patients.

Once you are clear that it is not your approach that is creating the problem, what should you do to elicit compliance?

- **Don't take the impasse personally**. To do so just adds problems to your relationship with them.
- **Clarify the message**. Be clear about what you each need to do now. Do not bring in previous examples of their noncompliance, such as "the last time this happened," or "you always," or "remember when you . . ." Focus on the immediate problem.
- **Stay on topic**. Do not allow the person to divert your attention to unrelated issues. Simply say, "Malik, we can talk about that later, but right now . . ."
- **Use a strong and calm voice**. Make your tone of voice strong but not forceful or aggressive.
- **De-personalize your role in the interactions**. Rather than saying, "Josiah, I expect you to . . ." try saying, "Josiah, you know you are expected to . . ." or "The rules of this hospital are . . ."
- **State the consequences**. Consequences are **NOT** punishments designed to break the other person's will or *make* him do what you want. Consequences should be provided as "information," rather than threats, the same way you inform someone on a cold winter day, "If you stick your tongue on that metal pole, you are going to get stuck." Or, in a situation germane to the hospital environment, "If you do not take your medications, you will have to talk about that today with your doctor."
- **Place the power in their hands**. Without handing over one iota of your authority, allow the patient to be the decision maker, clarifying their role in complying or not complying with your

request or directive. After summing up the situation, say something like, "It looks like you've got something to decide. You are absolutely correct. You don't have to do it. You can change your clothes and then we can go to the television room, or you can wear the same clothes and we won't. You will decide what's best for you now." If, at this point, you simply stand and look at him, it can be interpreted as a challenge, with you tapping your foot waiting for him to do what you want him to do. Instead, ease back, ease away, and give him some time to think. Perhaps you can say, "Let me know when you've made up your mind about what you want to do." Be sure to thank the person if he does comply.

Summary: Coping with stubborn refusals
- Do not take the impasse personally.
- Clarify the message.
- Stay on topic.
- Use a calm and strong voice.
- De-personalize your role.
- State the consequences.
- Place the power in their hands.

CHAPTER 5

Coping with Repetitive Demands,
Questions, and Obsessions

Sometimes your patients make repetitive demands for information that you have already answered or explained in exhaustive detail. There can be a variety of reasons for this, and each should be dealt with in a different manner:

They become "stuck" in an obsessive thought or idea. No matter how many times you answer their question, they have to ask it again. This is often a sign of obsessive-compulsive disorder (OCD), something frequently missed by evaluators because many patients become skilled in covering it up. It is important to help them get professional assistance specific to this disorder. In some cases, you will contact the proper mental health service provider yourself if they are unable to do so on their own.[1]

Others obsess as part of a disorder like schizophrenia, developmental disability, or other serious impairments of cognition. If they are re-asking the question because they either forgot or didn't understand the answer, it is most reasonable to answer them again. If they are not able to retain the information, please refer to the information in Chapter 3. These individuals are not playing games; they simply have cognitive deficits that cripple their ability to understand and/or retain information.

Sometimes people repeat a question *intending* to be irritating or challenging. In a bland tone of voice, simply say, "You already know the answer to that," or otherwise calmly point out that they already have the information, and *move on*, either physically or by changing the subject. If you linger after you respond, particularly while holding eye contact, it can be seen as a challenge, as if to say, "So how do you like my answer, huh?" By disengaging, you are saying, "I'm not participating in the game."

Sometimes the person is genuinely pleading for information, but what they really want to know is "behind" the question they are asking. For example, your patient might have asked, "When is my Uncle Harry coming?" five times already. You finally say, "You are really worried about this, even though I've told you he's coming at four o'clock. What's different about Uncle Harry's coming today?" Then, and not before, she reveals that yesterday she picked up her uncle's glasses to try them on, and she broke them. She is worried that her uncle will be mad when he arrives.

Sometimes, people *perseverate*, meaning they are stuck on a subject and feel like they have to talk about it. With certain patients, for whom this is a significant problem, say something like, "I know this is very important to you, and you want to talk about this and ask me questions. But you also know I have a lot of things to do. I will make you an agreement. We will talk about this for seven minutes every day. You can speak to me about this at exactly 2:15 p.m. But it will be seven minutes only. I will listen carefully and answer any questions you have, but you have to think hard and decide exactly what you want to talk about each day, because at the end of seven minutes, I'll say 'TIME,' and that's it for that day." It is essential that at the end of the imposed time limit, you firmly and definitely end the conversation or questioning for that day. Depending on your professional responsibilities and the situation, you can make two or three time periods a day with some people. What is most important, though, is to hold exactly to the time.

Example: Timing contacts with perseverating patients

A mental health professional found it quite helpful to put an egg timer on his desk, which he set to a specified time limit when he began his interview with certain patients. This established a definitive time frame for the interview and was rather effective in keeping some of his more disorganized patients focused on what was being discussed.

CHAPTER 6

The Need for Reassurance

Suffering from anxiety is living as if something that you are afraid might happen ***is happening right now,*** or living with feelings of imminent doom. For example, you read about an earthquake in Japan and imagine what might happen to your town if an earthquake hit, and suddenly, you feel as horrible as if the ground has started shaking right beneath your feet.

When working with someone afflicted by anxiety disorders, you must draw a graceful line. Despite what may be considerable sympathy that you have for them, do not coddle the person. If you treat them like they are too weak or frail for this world, they will possibly believe you. They may think that something awful is going to happen and that is why you are talking in such careful tones. If you are too dismissive of their fears, however, you will alienate them, making him feel that much more abandoned. Part of true reassurance is *assurance* that you will stand by them and help them face what they fear.

Working with someone afflicted with anxiety
- Do not treat them like they are fragile.
- Do not make your voice "overconfident" or "jovial" or in any other manner be dismissive of their concerns.
- Talk with them about their worries, using a confident voice that makes the person feel stronger for listening.

CHAPTER 7

Dealing with Individuals with
Pronounced Mood Swings

These individuals, whose behavior is sometimes referred to as labile, are angry one minute, sad the next, and happy the next. Those diagnosed with borderline personality disorder, bipolar disorder, or neurological damage, be it from traumatic brain injury or traumatic levels of drug abuse, often display labile modes.

Such patients can be very hard to communicate with, much less de-escalate, because as we try to deal with their current mood, they change just when we think we have achieved a moment of success.

They often try to gain control over us even when they have no control over themselves. They can be verbally abusive, provocative, complaining, passive-aggressive, blaming, apologetic, ingratiating, and friendly all in the space of an hour – or less.

Coping with Mood Swings

Rather than respond to the patient's momentary moods, either verbally or with body language that suggests your own anger or frustration, you must remain balanced and emotionally nonreactive (Section IV). The more you are unaffected by their emotional storms, the more you can influence them in a positive way. This is an "active" calm that provides a sense of safety and stability within the people around you.

Review: Mood swings
- Do not mirror their emotional state, or allow them to elicit from you an inappropriate emotional response.
- Remain powerfully calm.
- Speak in a firm yet calm and controlled manner.
- Use de-escalation tactics in this book to deal with expressions of aggression.

CHAPTER 8

Moving Past the Past

Some people store up grievances, and allow feelings of persecution and perceived personal slights to affect their entire worldview. These feelings can be more problematic with mentally ill patients, because their memories may be distorted or even delusional. Frequent complaints about old history can become a significant barrier to a patient's compliance with treatment, not to mention an aggravation to the harried treatment provider who must continually turn the patient's attention to the immediate issues and future concerns.

Unfortunately, you may represent the "last stop" along a patient's very long and very frustrating journey through the medical, social services, and mental health system(s), and they will often attempt to take out their frustrations, and address the indignities they feel they have suffered, on you.

As with disorganized (Chapter 14) and labile patients (Chapter 7), you must refrain from reacting emotionally to the patient's inability to move beyond the past, even as you try to redirect their attention to the present. Above all, do not personalize their complaints or their feelings of prior injustices. You can hardly be expected to bear the emotional burden for entire mental health or medical systems, or feel responsible for any previous mistreatment or improprieties surrounding the patient's case. How then can you deflect their accusations, and perhaps even alleviate their concerns?

Acknowledge their concerns. Quite often patients merely need to express their frustrations or feelings of helplessness about their situation, and they view you, as a representative of "the system," as the only available outlet to do so. Sometimes, allowing them to express their feelings (in an appropriate manner) and acknowledging their viewpoint is enough to alleviate their anger. Do not agree or disagree with them, or otherwise reinforce their feelings of persecution; just recognize their complaints and then move forward. <u>Do not, however, allow the patient to revisit the issue at every interview; strive to make this a "one and done" event</u>.

Apologize. When your patient complains, yet again, about something directly concerning you, think about it very carefully. Perhaps, in this instance, you were wrong. If so, apologize sincerely and fully. In some situations, this is enough. However, <u>you should be wary of apologizing to a patient merely as a means of moving them off a specific subject or grievance</u>. An apology may lead the patient to believe they are now in control of the relationship, and that you will act cautiously so you don't upset them in the future. To avoid this dilemma, act ethically and professionally at all times. By staying calm and in control you are much less likely to say or do anything for which you would need to apologize later.

What if an apology is not enough? Some people perseverate – they continue to bring up a complaint over and over again.

- You may say to the patient, "You are still upset about this. You want to talk about it again, don't you?" Notice that you don't ask the patient – you merely state your understanding. This is empowering, because they have the opportunity to correct or adjust your understanding. At the same time, you are probably right – and you thereby demonstrate that you understand them. As you will read below, this, alone, can have a very positive effect on your relationship with the patient.

- If you are aware that the patient has a legitimate, as yet unresolved complaint, firmly and kindly say, "Tomas, I said I am sorry and I meant it. I will never do anything like that again. You don't have to worry about that." From this point, you have a number of alternatives. One option is "paraphrasing" (Chapter 44) to try to ascertain if there is more that is disturbing your patient, because logically speaking, the proper response to a sincere apology is acceptance.

Complaints are their own reward. Certain people are never satisfied, because the complaint becomes a "rewarding" activity in itself. Others bear a pervasive resentment toward you, an institution, or even life itself. For them, complaints are merely a way to express hostility or an attempt to control the interview by getting you to talk about their agenda. In these cases, simply take the issue off the table, forever. Remind them that you have already addressed this complaint, so that there is nothing more to discuss.

Review: Moving past the past

1. Acknowledge their concerns.
2. Apologize.
3. When patients are stuck on an issue
   - Validate the patient's continued distress.
   - Reiterate a necessary apology, emphatically, with reassurance.
4. When complaints are their own reward, set a firm limit and take the issue "off the table."

CHAPTER 9

"Would You Just Get off Your Rear End?": Coping with Lack of Motivation

You've surely been in situations where you ask or even tell a mentally ill patient to do something, and they stare vacantly at you, voice a million questions, express misgivings or anxiety, or drift into a monologue about something completely different. Other mentally ill patients seem to lack motivation; they just won't do those things we believe are necessary for their own well-being.

In such cases, you must ask yourself if the patient is truly capable of doing what you think he should, or if they even understand what you are asking. You may want him to participate in a group meeting, but he suffers from terrible social anxiety and being so close to other people is misery. He may be happier alone, and, in fact, will do better in the hospital if allowed to do so. This may not be the life you desire for your patient, but this is who he is.

You must also ask yourself if what you want him to do is really important. Your patient would look so much nicer if he wore different clothes, but he doesn't see it that way. He says he hates the feel of certain material on his hypersensitive skin, and he doesn't want to look handsome anyway. Perhaps he is afraid that if he is thought to be handsome, strange women will bother or sexually harass him. Or perhaps he feels terribly unsafe when he goes out of the home – yet he bravely does that every day so that he can go to his place of employment. Added attention might make him feel so uneasy that he will quit his job.

On the other hand, if you do for your patients what they could do for themselves, they may become quite comfortable in their dependency. It is an easy life when someone takes care of you. You must also be honest in evaluating whether they indeed can do something. If you don't protect them, they may suffer the consequences of their inaction, but there is also the possibility that they will have to take responsibility for things they can do.

Finally, you should take note of just how you attempt to motivate your patient. Do you like the sound of your voice? Are you pleading, whining, nagging, yelling, or making other unattractive sounds? You should offer advice in a firm tone of voice, and neither hover nor sound like a "cheerleader" in an attempt to get them to comply. When you are dignified, your patients will respect you more, sometimes in spite of themselves. People are far more likely accept advice from a person they respect.

Review: Coping with a patient's lack of motivation
- Ascertain if they are capable of complying with your request or directive.
- Is it really important?
- Do not do for others what they can do for themselves.
- Have you lost your dignity in the way that you are trying to get them to comply? Act in a manner that merits respect.

CHAPTER 10

"If There Is a Problem, That Would Be Your Fault": Useful Tactics for Dealing with Symptoms of Paranoia and Persecution

This chapter focuses on tactics specific to a paranoid attitude.
Rather than the delusional state (Chapters 17 and 18), this discussion will focus on an attitude: a sense of being persecuted, blame of others for any problem, and a hair-trigger sensitivity to being vulnerable. The delusional paranoid individual has this attitude complicated by fixed false beliefs and even hallucinations.

Understanding Paranoia and Persecution

A sense of persecution is only part of the paranoid dilemma. The paranoid world is an amalgam of dominance and submission. The paranoid individual often tries to dominate other people in their lives, and all the while they are terrified or enraged at being forced to submit. This is a very primitive defense mechanism that can be summed up like this: "If there is a problem here, that would be your fault."

When we speak of paranoia, we are referring not only to a psychotic or delusional state, but also to the far more common paranoid character, in which the person has a consistent *attitude* of blame, resentment of authority, fear of vulnerability, and expectations of betrayal.

People experiencing paranoia are, at core level, very frightened, but they cover this up with suspicion and aggression. Paranoid people are "counter-phobic" – they are aggressive toward that of which they are afraid. Imagine your patient like a big, angry porcupine. They feel excruciatingly vulnerable: they have no quills on their underside, so to speak, so they try to keep their backs to you all the time, hunched over and ready to strike in hair-trigger reaction.

One thing that makes us feel most vulnerable is love and affection. Paranoid people, however, experience love, evoking feelings of vulnerability, as an attack. For this reason, paranoid people are particularly volatile within their families.

Rapport, which should make things easier, is a problematic factor in working with paranoid patients. When they feel any comfort with you, they also recoil, because loving feelings of affection or trust might make them vulnerable. You should, therefore, be prepared for the patient to suddenly act out with suspicion or accusations during times that are uneventful or even, within professional limits, friendly. For this person, it is as if their quills, the paranoid defenses that they believe keep them safe, are softening as they relax.

Being mistaken or wrong is another form of vulnerability. Because these patients will not admit to wrongdoing or mistakes, they automatically ***project*** negative feelings onto the other person. If, for example, they feel hate, they believe, "You hate me." If they have difficulty in understanding an application for public assistance, they say, "I wouldn't have messed it up if it hadn't been for you. I shouldn't have trusted you."

These individuals live in their own world like detectives, searching for clues and evidence to prove what they already know is true. They may have ***ideas of reference***, in which they believe that other's conversations, glances, or actions are directed at them, and no amount of arguing will dissuade them. They assume that others are probably conspiring about them, talking about them, and laughing at them; and their actions, in response to this belief, often evoke the behavior they fear.

When people in paranoid states are afraid, they often attack, either verbally or physically. Even without an overt attack, they frequently make other people uncomfortable because of their aggressive or standoffish behavior. However, if they sense fear in you, due to the emotions they have evoked with their own behavior, they expect you to attack, and they will then "attack you back first." It is very important, therefore, to master your anxiety and fear so that you do not betray your feelings with trembling hands, a shaking voice, or an inability to hold eye contact. Perhaps the most valuable method to accomplish this is through proper breathing methods (Chapter 24).

Try to Let Them Know What Is Going On

Because these patients are so suspicious, they will often question your actions and instructions. Although you would do this with any other patient, it is particularly important to clearly and explicitly explain the rules and regulations of the hospital and why you are doing something. Whenever you can, tell them what you are doing. Better yet, show them:

> *"Arnie, I was writing my chart notes. See. Here's your name. And here are the notes. 'Med refill in two weeks, follow-up appointment with the nurse for your infected foot.' I was just about to write the address for your new financial worker at the DSHS office. Could you repeat that to me so I don't make any mistakes?"*

At the same time, you should not accept being quizzed incessantly. You are not required to explain every action. You will have to learn to strike a balance. Sometimes it is quite right to simply say, "Kent, I've answered enough questions today," or, "Mrs. Adamson, I've told you everything I know."

Personal Space – Physical and Psychological – with the Paranoid Individual

Paranoid individuals feel safest when you differentiate yourself from them, so that you are not interwoven in their delusional fears. A more distant, even slightly impersonal, relationship is preferable to one that appears to be warm and friendly. Essentially, you imagine yourself in a dance – like a waltz, without contact – three arm's lengths apart. The "correct distance" is one that does not unnecessarily trigger fear and anger. Of course, a paranoid person can get lonely, just like any other individual. It is your responsibility, however, to maintain the "space," stepping back metaphorically or physically, as the situation demands, when they get too close. This is better, in the long run, than trying to seize an opportunity when their guard seems down to make your relationship "closer."

Many individuals with paranoia are preoccupied, even obsessed, with fears that they will be invaded, violated, or controlled in some fashion. Some find most physical contact, particularly that which is unsolicited, to be noxious. Because of these fears, personal spacing issues are important, particularly for the safety of staff and other patients.

- **Maintain the angle**. Particularly when sitting, turn your body at a slight angle, so that physical "confrontation" is a choice rather than a requirement. If you face a paranoid individual directly, you force *them* to turn away if he or she doesn't want to face you. This is true whether you are standing or sitting.
- **Never let your guard down**. This does not require *you* to be at hair-trigger readiness. However, never "take your ease" with a paranoid patient. Rather, stay calm and alert.
- **Too close is as dangerous as a threat**. Try to be aware when things are getting too relaxed. You may not be able to stop the patient's sudden anger, but it should not be unexpected.
- **Be aware of triggers that activate their paranoia**. There may be situations that activate the person's paranoia, those that bring up old resentments or are over-stimulating or exciting. Alcohol can make things worse as well.

Paranoid Aggression

There is not a specific "paranoid rage." Instead, paranoia is an engine that drives rage in all its various forms. Paranoid patients can exhibit fear, frustration, intimidation, and manipulation. When such an individual gets in a state of rage (Section IX) you will de-escalate them using tactics specific to the mode of rage they are exhibiting, rather than de-escalate "paranoia" itself.

Some disorganized people can experience an "omni-directional dread," an inchoate terror that is inescapable. In this case, you will de-escalate them using the principles regarding the disorganized patient (Chapters 14 and 57).

Review: Paranoia and persecution

The paranoid person has an attitude that anything wrong is another person's fault. Whether they are delusional or experiencing a manifestation of a fixed character trait, paranoid people see others as conspiring against them or persecuting them. They perceive any sense of vulnerability – even the ease of friendship or rapport – as dangerous.

- Use all the standard tactics for delusional people (Chapter 18) when speaking with paranoid patients.
- Let them know what's going on.
- Speak in somewhat formal tones.
- Avoid emotional and emotive language.
- Be aware of both physical and emotional spacing. Maintain a "correct distance" – not too close or too far.
- Stay centered: both calm and strong. The paranoid person is usually assaultive when they feel under attack, when they perceive you as controlling them, or when they sense that you are afraid.

SECTION II

A Consideration of Patients Whose Behaviors Make Them Particularly Difficult to Maintain in Inpatient Units

CHAPTER 11

Borderline Personality Disorder:
Treatment in Short-term Psychiatric Facilities
and Inpatient Crisis Units

Borderline personality disorder, like any pathological character trait, is a spectrum disorder, an accentuation of qualities common to all humanity. Any of us can be swept by feelings that seem beyond our control. Any of us can act on feelings that result in our making decisions that are not in our best interest, that may even be damaging to ourselves and others. Sometimes we are impulsive, and sometimes we get angry, even enraged. This alone is not the definition of borderline personality disorder.

The particular dilemma of borderline individuals is that they live in an existential universe: whatever they feel right now is their only reality. What for us are remarkable episodes in a usually calm and focused life are everyday occurrences for the person with borderline personality. Those on the mild end of the spectrum will be quite emotional, overreacting to events that others could take in stride. For those whose disorder is more severe, it is as if their nervous system – at least that which modulates emotion – lacks any protective sheathing. Imagine trying to live your daily life with two layers of skin peeled off. Any mundane experience could bring agony.

When life is felt with such exquisite force, one's current emotions are inescapable. One manifestation of this is an "allergy to ambiguity." They see the world and the people in it as good and bad, perfect and foul. The person who has such character traits lives with the passion, but also with the lack of emotional resilience, like that of a toddler.

A Discussion of Sexual Abuse as It Pertains to Those with Borderline Personality Disorder

There is considerable evidence that the development of borderline personality disorder is due to a combination of emotional sensitivity (basic disposition) and an abusive/chaotic upbringing. They have very frequently experienced sexual and/or physical abuse as children. It is unknown if the abuse is a precipitant of the development of borderline character traits, or if the prevalence of abuse histories among such patients is due to predatory individuals seeking out already emotionally sensitive children.

Victims of abuse, particularly those with borderline traits, may frequently raise the subject of their abuse history. Some patients may have learned to use it as a tragic strategy to get some power in interpersonal relationships because people will "back off" when the subject is raised. For example, a psych tech who tries to set a limit with a patient may feel abusive when the patient cries and accuses her of being just like her father.

Most people, however, are not manipulative, even unconsciously. However, they may have been taught, as part of therapy, to speak about what they have learned is the source of their psychological distress and to explain why they are acting or feeling the way they do. Many people rush to comfort the person when they raise their history of abuse, particularly if they do so with strong emotions. Please recall that the individual with borderline character traits lives in the present moment. Therefore, whatever they feel right now is most important to them. This means that their abuse history may become a way of eliciting comfort. The problem, however, is that nothing is healed: their "wound" is merely reopened, and later, once the comforting person has left to attend to other tasks, the person may feel raw and exposed, or worry that the staff person will hold them in contempt or will reveal their information to anyone they choose. They then go into a crisis; perhaps they will even become suicidal.

For this reason, the issue of abuse requires sensitivity:

Report current abuse. If a patient reveals current abuse, then staff must, of course, follow protocols to ensure their safety and report the situation to the proper authorities, as necessary.

Stay in your lane. Staff need to be very clear on their professional responsibilities. If a patient decides that a staff person is trustworthy and for the first time reveals a history of physical or sexual abuse, the staff person should listen with caring and respect, long enough to understand, in general terms, what happened to the person. If the staff person does not have direct responsibility as a therapist for the patient, they should gently intercede, and tell the person that they have the utmost respect for the courage it must have taken to reveal this information. However, the staff person must further explain that it is important that they receive help from someone who is trained to give such therapeutic assistance. The next step would be to arrange for an appointment with a therapist properly trained in abuse issues, either on staff or as an outpatient referral. (Further details are contingent on the protocols of your hospital.)

When to engage in working on abuse issues. Of course, if you are the proper person to work with the person, both by training and role, then you should engage in therapeutic work. However, this, too, needs to be properly titrated, particularly if the person's hospital stay is short-term. Don't start something you cannot finish! Perhaps you will be able to arrive at an interim place in treatment and properly transition them to outpatient work.

Get a release of information. If the person has an outpatient therapist, hospital staff should endeavor to get a release of information, and follow the outpatient therapist's guidance on how best to make use of the patient's time while in the hospital. It is quite possible that the therapist will recommend that staff tell the patient that these are issues best discussed with their therapist upon their discharge from the hospital, and your response should be confined to, "And while you are here, we will focus on . . ."

Help the patient to develop a sense of privacy. If the patient repetitively or compulsively raises the subject, particularly with varied people, staff must be trained to say, "That is very personal information.

I am not trained to help you with that, and anyway, you are working on that with your therapist." On some occasions, I recommend that the staff person point out that in the past, when the patient has openly discussed abuse issues, they have subsequently spiraled into another crisis. One aspect of psychological health is a sense of privacy and proportion: this is particularly important for people who react so dramatically to negative emotions.

In maintaining the proper boundary in regards to this deeply painful history, you are showing the patient one of the finest human traits: tact. If it is not your business, or if you do not have the training to know how to respond to their account, the kindest thing is to (a) redirect them to their treatment plan and what they can accomplish in the hospital, and (b) guide them to people who can best help them, in a way that does not compromise either their overall treatment plan or their stay in the hospital.

Splitting

Because of this combination of character traits, individuals with borderline personality disorder frequently find themselves in various crises. Among them are suicidal attempts; parasuicidal acts (self-mutilating behaviors or repeat suicide "attempts" that were either gestures for effect or staged in a manner that despite the seriousness of the act, are found out; see Chapters 32 and 33); impulsive assaultive acts, particularly those involving family or other close relationships; and brief psychotic episodes. In essence, such a person believes that whatever feeling they are having right now is the only possible reality. For example, road rage is a borderline reaction: someone cuts a person off, it makes them mad, and instead of cooling down, they chase after them and smash into their car. On the flip side, they meet someone attractive in a bar, and within five seconds, they know that this is the love of their life.

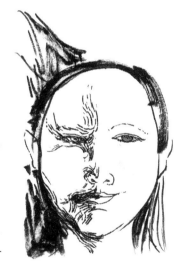

In reaction to the dramatic and emergent events that so frequently occur in such individual's lives, many of the people associated with the patient, including their outpatient therapist(s), disagree about the most appropriate treatment course of action, even to the point of arguing about who is at fault for the patient's current crisis. Those involved in a therapeutic relationship with the patient often contextualize, explain, or excuse the behavior, especially when they have a previous history of trauma or abuse. When the individuals associated with a borderline person get tangled up in intense disputes about what is best for them, this type of conflict is called *splitting*.

The patient, although not entirely conscious of what they are doing, is at the center of the conflict, but it doesn't occur in a vacuum. You are also an integral part of it. Splitting should be regarded as a tactic in which the patient presents a different facet of their personality to each person with whom they interact. This "divide and confuse" strategy often sets family members, treatment providers, social services personnel, and legal system representatives against one another regarding the proper response to the patient's behavior. It is a primitive defense mechanism that the individual develops in hopes of "disappearing": through engendering conflict, the significant figures in their life can never unite to focus on them. If one has an early history of chaos and abuse, such a strategy may provide a modicum of safety, at least compared to what might happen if everyone unified to negatively focus on them.

Although splitting is usually regarded as an "action" by the patient, one that is, at best, unconsciously manipulative and, at worst, sociopathic, this is too simplistic. Splitting is a process, not an act. Professionals are also participants in splitting, and quite frankly, sometimes the actions of these professionals *create* the splitting process. Not surprisingly, patients with borderline personality disorder will appear quite different to a therapist trying to build a supportive, non-confrontational relationship than to a psych tech or hospital social worker trying to help them negotiate their way through day-to-day life in the hospital, and a probation officer, who is most responsible for public safety and who can quickly take away the patient's freedom. Needless to say, each responds to the patient somewhat differently, and each may believe that they have the best idea on how to deal with them. Unfortunately, these varying opinions, and not coincidentally, a measure of professional pride, can lead to arguments about the best course of action.

In cases such as these, one or another party may decide to unilaterally make a decision based on what they believe is the patient's best interest. However, if all members of the defacto team responsible for the patient remain at odds, the "victory" by the person who made the unilateral decision will be short-lived. You will be working with the same people on other cases, and you will most likely continue to be "at odds/together" regarding this patient. Thus, whenever intense conflict or a divergence of opinions regarding a single patient arises, suggest the possibility of splitting and see if you can, by comparing observations, determine if the patient's interactions with various people have created the adversarial situation. The patient's case should be respectfully discussed among the treatment team to flesh out any necessary changes to the treatment plan. Without such consultation, an incredible amount of time and effort can be spent arguing about the status of one patient.

None of the above minimizes the seriousness of this character disorder or the genuine anguish that individuals suffer. At the same time, inappropriate or ineffective treatment, offered with the best intentions in the world, is not helpful. The following sequence is common:
- The individual presents in severe crisis, necessitating law enforcement and/or mental health professionals to intervene.
- They are taken to an inpatient unit. Often, after a period of resistance – which can include suicide attempts and assaultive or disruptive behaviors – the individual adjusts to the milieu.
- They are still seen as fragile, and this viewpoint is substantiated as treatment professionals interview the person. Issues of current or past abuse come up, and the person with the borderline disorder becomes emotionally volatile – with frequent mood swings, associated with "what comes up in therapy or group discussions."
- The patient becomes increasingly bonded to some practitioners, or even to the unit itself. In a very short time, it becomes a family system to them. As is typical with such individuals, they

may idealize one or another staff or patient, wanting to spend as much time as possible with them. Their need becomes consuming. At the same time, they may form a negative transference with other staff. This negativity is not mere dislike. In their all or nothing world, they idealize and they hate.

- Given that borderline splitting is an unconscious process, not only do staff evoke feelings simply by virtue of interacting with them, but also the borderline person may associate such feelings with images of family members or other people significant in their lives. Such feelings can be multilayered. The longer a borderline patient is in an inpatient unit, the more such feelings will be evoked. Splitting can be productively worked on in long-term therapy, where a patient is taught to become aware of their unconscious reactions and fantasies. But short-term inpatient facilities (drug-treatment or emergency hospitals) are not the places to do this family systems work.

Example: Borderline splitting with a patient

Samantha, a case manager, reminds the patient of her mother, whom she loved. She is, therefore, enraged with her because she never successfully stopped the abuse she suffered at the hands of her father. Eleni somehow reminds the patient of her second-grade schoolteacher, whom she disliked and who disliked her. It is equally possible that the patient is oppositional and aggressive to Eleni, or in an unconscious attempt to "do better this time," she is ingratiating and compliant.

- Problems frequently arise around discharge planning. Some staff may grow increasingly concerned because of the patient's volatility there is increasing fear that if the patient is released, they will come to harm, either by their own hand, or due to their interactions with others. If such discharge planning is brought up to the patient, they may become enraged – feeling rejected by their "family," and also cut off from those in the unit for whom they may have formed intense feelings. In some cases, they may be in the unit for months – with no improvement whatsoever in their basic level of functioning.
- Finally, familiarity breeds contempt. Staff are seen as toxic family members, jailers, or rejecting love objects. The end result is a pernicious cycle that culminates in assaults – sometimes very serious – on staff or other patients, serious suicide attempts, or a flare up of self-mutilating behaviors.

It is fair to say that in such a situation, the treatment facility has become a vector of psychological pathology. Without any ill intent, the hospital and its members constellate the behaviors that, clinically, we would hope to alleviate.

A Solution

Inpatient intervention for borderline personality disorder requires several components.

As this is a disorder of emotions, the intervention must focus on these areas. If a child receives the greatest amount of attention for negative behavior, he or she will increase those behaviors. It is the same for the individual with borderline character traits. Whenever the individual is disruptive and "acting out," interactions with staff should have some warmth, but should also be phlegmatic and brief. The patient's safety should be ensured, but verbal and emotional interactions should be short and "dry."

Given that borderline patients are quite reactive to other people's emotional reactions, staff's attitude should be similar to that of a perfect uncle or aunt. In undeviatingly enforcing the rules and paying attention to what is really going on, you are definitely an authority; but because you maintain a degree of emotional "distance," you don't get emotionally worked up.

An essential component of treatment is to assist the patient in managing the tension-relaxation cycle. It is not enough to teach the patient relaxation or stress-reduction exercises. One way to think of the borderline dilemma is to imagine an overtired child who "cannot settle." As they get tense, they feel like they will explode, but if they relax, they feel like they will fly apart. Therefore, the patient must be taught procedures that involve both the body and the breath, which give them a sense of control over their psycho-physical states, so that they can relax when tense *and* give themselves some tension (tensile strength) when overly loose or relaxed.[2]

Participation in activities on the unit – groups, recreation, and so on – is contingent on good behavior. As the patient begins to show mature behavior, emotional interactions with staff should increase, typified by warmth and approval.

Discharge planning should be initiated upon <u>entry</u>. With repeat patients who have numerous psychiatric emergencies, a wrap-around plan with outpatient services should be triggered upon entry.

The patient should be discharged as soon as they are stabilized. This can be as brief as a matter of hours or only a few days. Cure cannot happen within the inpatient unit. Improvement, even cure in some cases, occurs through enrollment in a comprehensive therapeutic program. In such cases, the inpatient unit functions as a crisis respite bed when the patient gets in situations that he or she cannot manage "outside." If the individual is kept at the hospital beyond stabilization, they will, as described above, begin to express their pathological style in reaction to the milieu. Rather than a respite, the hospital and its staff will become the triggers for new crises.

An effective program integrates the hospital as part of the treatment program. Therefore, individuals with borderline personality traits who are new to your local mental health system need to be enrolled, whenever possible, in an effective treatment program that is willing to work, hand-in-glove, with the hospital.

If your hospital program is too comfortable and "homelike," patients will make themselves "at home." Short-term respite units should be clean and well run, but not a place to make a nest. For example, I'm aware of some units where one sleeps in a comfortable easy chair rather than a bed. The message, given with kindness, is, "Don't make yourself at home."

You must be prepared for some patients to "flare" when they are treated differently than they may desire ("I'm upset and you are not comforting me!" is one example). They may escalate their behaviors, sometimes in very dangerous ways. Staff must be prepared for this. A hospital that cannot manage a borderline patient's disruptive, assaultive, or destructive behaviors cannot adequately serve such patients anyway. Colluding with the patient's pathological style is not therapy and will not help. Just as with a child who is used to getting what they want through public tantrums, borderline patients must be consistently treated with matter-of-fact strong discipline. Staff must maintain the protocols, even if some patients try to undermine them through an increase of pathological behaviors. Although the patient in the middle of his or her emotional storm may not agree, kindness and ethics are both best served when staff act in a way that will, in the long run, help the patient manage those storms better.

Even individuals who refuse to participate in an outpatient program should be subject to a protocol that includes the principles I have outlined. Such a protocol offers the patient the best hope that, in the future, they will engage in comprehensive services. It must be noted that this – alone – is *not* a protocol. I am merely describing some of the principles required in setting up a protocol.

Among "best practice" for those with borderline personality disorder is Dialectical-Behavioral Therapy (DBT), pioneered by Dr. Marsha Linehan of the University of Washington. Inpatient units that work with those with borderline personality would do well to consult with Dr. Linehan or another professional (or psychiatric hospital) fully trained in DBT methods.

Review: Working with those with borderline traits and dealing with splitting

- Stay focused on whether or not there is really an emergent issue.
- Do not be reactive to complaints or side issues the person brings up. Reward positive behaviors and deal with negative behaviors with an absolute minimum of emotion (thereby offering no reward). From your side, your emotional interaction should exemplify "warm distance."
- When abuse issues are raised, "stay in your lane." If you are not a therapist directly involved in their care, tactfully redirect them to their therapist – or work to help them get a therapist, who can actually assist them with this painful issue.
- Initiate discharge planning on admission.
- If they are a frequent admit to your hospital (or a resident in a group living situation), you will likely find yourself in a case that brings in players from many different systems and agencies; you must pool resources to arrive at a common viewpoint and plan for the patient.

CHAPTER 12

Bad Intentions: Recognizing the Strategies of Opportunistic and Manipulative Patients

Some people do not mean us well. They view us as opportunities to gain something they want, or animated toys to play with for their own amusement. Others live for hate and destruction, and delight most in duping people so that they do not even know how "dirty they were done." Others do not even *intend* to do harm; they are merely trying to survive. Based on a lifetime of negative experience, however, the best survival strategy they have ever been able to come up with entails lying and manipulation so that they aren't "caught." They use splitting (Chapter 11), a "divide and disappear" strategy, so that the more powerful beings in their life argue about them, thereby focusing on their newly created animosity toward each other rather than on the manipulative individual.

A Compendium of Manipulative Strategies[3]

Manipulative strategies are as varied as malevolence, desperation, and/or human creativity can devise. Let us consider the following:

Reframing: making something bad acceptable. One of the bitter truths in the helping professions is that we are often no better than lay people in detecting lying or manipulation. Once an alliance has been established (or so the staff person believes), professionals tend to give their patients the benefit of the doubt. Some professionals rationalize when they become aware of their patient doing something against the rules, reframing it not as malevolent or manipulative, but somehow "reasonable," because of their diagnosis, history, or whatever other context they impose to make the patient's actions somehow understandable. The manipulative patient assesses the professional in his or her "interview" process, tracking their reactions to ascertain what will evoke the most sympathy or protective reaction on the part of the professional so that they begin to engage in reframing.

Example: Reframing creating danger

One of the support staff at your hospital states that she is uneasy around a patient. He is an often angry young man who has complained bitterly about how older women treat him, that they clutch their purse or lock their car doors when they see him "just because I'm of (X culture), or dressed like (fill in the blank)." After a fair amount of time and a lot of hard work, he seems to trust you, one of those older women who has otherwise caused him such distress. He has a beautiful smile that the world is graced with all too rarely, and he tells you, "You are cool. You understand where I'm coming from." So you discount the support staff person's complaint, attributing it to prejudice or social rigidity (she's not "cool" like you). However, the truth is that this young man runs his eyes over her body and leans over the front desk. In fact, he is engaged in the beginnings of predatory stalking – assessing if this woman is viable as prey.

Putting you on the spot. Manipulative people put you on the spot by asking for a decision in front of others (family members, for example) where your refusal will cause disappointment or distress.

Example: Putting staff on the spot

While holding her son's hand, a woman says to a nurse responsible for supervising her court-mandated visits: "You know, I promised my son that we'd celebrate his birthday party here. It's his seventh birthday. It won't hurt if he sees me, his mother, for just few extra hours. It's his birthday, after all."

Telling lies of omission. Often dishonesty is manifested as a lie of omission. They will tell you reassuring aspects of a situation but not include their intention to harm.

Example: Lie of Omission

Safety protocols dictate that two staff persons are required to go into patients' rooms in a certain ward. As you wait for your teammate, the patient says, "My roommate's here. She's cool. I guess you are a little uncomfortable going into a person's room by yourself. Don't worry. I'm not like the other people in this program." Notice that the person has given you no promise that they will not harm you.

Making reassuring promises. One sign of coercion is a reassuring promise when none was asked for. For example: "I know you might be concerned. I only need to talk with you for five minutes, I promise."

Giving too much information. One way to manage the perceptions of others is to talk too much, too elaborately. The manipulative person uses charm to keep their victim's attention focused on the relationship, or on the fascinating details of their stories, rather than on what they are doing. In so doing, when an issue of concern arises, the manipulative person tries to get you to "contextualize" those concerns in his or her favor.

Example: Too much information

You are interviewing a man about his past, and you ask him for a sexual history. He laughs and says, "That's really not a concern any more. I admit, twenty years ago, that would have been a relevant question. I had lots of lovers, men and women. I came in at the tail end of the glam-rock scene, and I had some times!" He tells you an outrageously entertaining story about a famous entertainer, a limo, two bottles of Armagnac, and a bucket of prune whip Danish. Then he tells you a second story, more outrageous than the last. As you try to get back on track, he says, "But I've been celibate – I guess you'd call it – for about ten years. I don't function any more, and to tell you the truth, I'm not interested. I know there are pills these days, but I've started meditating, and I'd rather be doing that than medicating." You are charmed and entertained, and end up not asking details about his sexual activities over this ten-year period, taking his "not functioning" at face value.

However, many men's sex lives do not end just because they no longer "function." He doesn't "have sex" any more than a certain ex-president didn't "have sex with that woman." In the case of our charming ex-rock star, he molests his own children, something he doesn't consider "sex" because "they are family." But he is now on record with his doctor as being "impotent" and "uninterested." The danger now is that others who review his records may not pay attention to warning signs of abuse that otherwise would be noticed during the children's visits to the hospital.

Gathering your personal information. The manipulative person will ask for personal information. This is not only intimate information, but also everyday stuff. For many readers, there is a certain level of basic information that is not of concern whatsoever. What is off-limits is determined by your job responsibilities and who your patients are. Nonetheless, information can become leverage. The manipulator can use this information to further conversational topics, to "find" points in common, and, thereby, to enlist you in a positive view of them. Sometimes, the manipulative person will use the information to make it look like you have a special or intimate relationship.

Example: Using personal information

A patient in a group session says in a low voice, as if trying to keep something private, yet clearly in earshot of other group members, "Hey Jennifer, how's your car doing? Did you take my advice about changing your timing belt?" The manipulative person is able to make it appear that they are good friends, diminishing the staff person's authority in the eyes of both patients and other staff.

Blackmailing through information acquisition. Manipulators also strive to acquire information that the staff person would not want revealed. The staff person is informed by the patient just what that information is. In the interest of avoiding embarrassment, the staff person may then give in to patient's demands. At a certain point, these requests become illegal or unethical, and the staff member can be blackmailed. *Any innocuous question, even what kind of car you drive or what brand of beer you might drink, is leverage.* I am not saying you must be totally closed off, but be mindful what you are revealing, to whom, and what possible "blowback" there might be. Forensic patients, in particular, are always attempting to listen to staff communication, thereby overhearing personal information.

Example: Use of information for blackmail or predatory attack

You are in a lunch area and mention that your wife has a "girl's night out" on Wednesdays. You add that she saw a certain music group that she really liked and this club, she tells you, is a great place. You don't like to dance, so you don't go with her, but you don't worry, because no one hassles the women, the music is good, and the drinks are cheap. You are over-heard. It will take only a few inquiries by a resourceful individual to find out that Roomful of Blues, the group in question, was playing at the Cosmo Club. The possibilities at this point are wide open. Either the forensic patient, when he is released, or someone he calls today, may pay a visit to the club one Wednesday night, and he observes your wife using an illegal drug. You are now open to blackmail. And that is not the worst possibility: instead of merely observing, this charming, roguish man approaches to ask for a . . . dance.

Assessing behavior. Manipulative people make many behavioral observations. They are particularly interested in who is intimidated, easily frightened, or overly macho. All of these are "off-center postures." People who are off-center are easy to manipulate, physically or emotionally, because they are easily "moved."

Example: Using behavioral assessment to divide and conquer

The psych tech associated with a patient is a no-nonsense type who sticks to the rules. The manipulative individual notices another psych tech who is off-center, perhaps a little shy and easily intimidated. The patient will try to set in motion a case transfer so that they can "work" with a person who is easier to intimidate or otherwise control.

Spurious rescuing. Manipulative people sometimes wait for a situation where a staff person is victimized by a patient, so the manipulator can rescue them. Some manipulators simply wait for an opportune moment. Others stage the event from start to finish.

Example: Fake rescue

In a long-term inpatient unit, or a group home for aggressive youth, a resident might pick out a new staff member and offer to show them "the ropes." The resident might adopt a protective air or have another resident stage an aggressive act, even an attack, from which the first resident will be the rescuer. "Hey, he's cool! Stop talking like that, man!" Then later, "Mr. Edmondson, I'm sorry about James. He's got a bad attitude. Look, I know you are new here – I do not mean any disrespect – it's just that you don't know who's who and what's what yet. If you have any questions, you ask me. And you don't have to worry about James. I told him you are cool."

Quid pro quo. We are social beings, and, therefore, our relationships are based, in part, on mutual exchange. If people do us a favor, we often feel like we owe them. Manipulative people deliberately do favors to set up an opportunity for a demand in return. One way they accomplish this is through flattery: "Wow, how did you get that about me? I feel like you translate things so my husband can understand what I'm saying."

Another type of favor is simpler. I recall another example where a patient insisted in lending a paraprofessional five dollars because she had forgotten her bus pass. She attempted to pay him back the next day, but he refused, making an issue out of it. "My money's too good for you? Can't a man do someone a favor? Why are you treating me like some kind of crazy person? If we were friends, you would accept my gift."

Another way of setting up a quid pro quo is "making it difficult." Many manipulators frame openness in social services as a favor. By deliberately making it very hard to get information or work with them, and *then* offering information that was long awaited, they may actually be trying to set up some kind of return favor that they claim (and might believe) that they are owed.

It may be hard to accept that you are being manipulated

After all, you do your work with the intention of helping the vulnerable and the disabled achieve a better life. For the manipulative person, however, your job is a scam: you get people to tell you things or comply with certain behaviors so that you can get paid. Therefore, their openness is part of transaction. Implicit is a message: "By telling you this, I'm helping you get paid. Now what are you going to give me in return? In fact, you owe me now."

You're the boss. Another tactic is "conceding" that the staff person is the decision maker, the powerful one.

Example: You're the boss

"Hey, you call the shots, ma'am. You decide. That's actually why I'm asking. Is there any chance I could see you tomorrow so that you could explain this paperwork to me? I appreciate that you don't have time today, but some of these words are a little difficult for me, so I wondered if you had some extra time . . ."

Accompanying such obsequiousness, such individuals can be "accident-prone." They frequently "accidentally" undermine tasks or responsibilities.

- "Gee, it broke. I am SO sorry!"
- "I did try to get to the doctor's office. You don't think I wanted to have my car break down, do you? Now I have to wait six weeks for another appointment! I cannot believe you are blaming me for a mechanical failure, like I knew I'd get a flat."

Attacking leverage points. The manipulator will attack you not only through your weak points, but also through your best points. The manipulator scans his or her victim looking for leverage – anything, strong or weak, that they can use.

Examples: Leverage points

- If you are religious, you very likely have a faith in the redemption of people. A patient's showing contrition for a crime or other hurtful act, even if he or she makes no religious references whatsoever, may lead you to let down your guard. Guess who knew you went to church?
- Let us say that one of your proudest attributes is your willingness to help the underdog or the oppressed. The manipulator will "become" a victim of oppression, and then, when other people have caught him doing something out of line, you will, believing what you were set up to believe, defend the person who is, once again, being unfairly "victimized."

Grooming. The manipulative person may set up a situation where he creates in you a little anxiety and then relieves it *while making a request you would have granted anyway.*

Grooming behavior

He stands too close – just a little – and then, as he pulls back, he asks for a drink of water. Similar actions will be repeated until the "target" begins to associate a sense of relief and relaxation *when they are granting a favor.* This can escalate until the favors are over an ethical or professional line. Groomed victims may rationalize this, because they are so used to feeling very good when granting favors to the person. Once the line has been crossed, however, it is too late. You are now "owned" by the other person.

> If this ever happens to you, you have only one way of saving yourself. Go immediately to your supervisor, and tell him or her how you have been compromised. In many cases, you will be criticized for your action and praised for your moral courage in coming forward, and with suitable corrective actions, will be able to keep your job. In other events, regrettably, you will be fired. But, in either event, if you do not "step up," you will become the slave of another person, forced to do things, criminal or unethical, against all your personal values.

Rumor-mongering and conscious splitting. Manipulators *consciously* split by spreading rumors or stories about other staff or patients. This may be lies, but it is even more effective when it's true. On other occasions, the manipulative individual will deliberately play one staff person against another, using everything from subtle cues in body language and facial expression to open favoritism toward one staff person and contempt toward another. (This is different from the more or less unconscious splitting that is described in Chapter 11. You need to distinguish between the two in order to adequately assess such factors as risk, your patient's intention, and how best to intervene. Staff need to discuss such behavior in detail to adequately determine if your patient is engaged in a calculated strategy or if it is more or less unconscious.)

Examples: Conscious splitting
- "Ms. Applegate, can I talk with you? You told me when I came here that staff worked hard to make this a safe place. Um, I don't know exactly how to say this, but I was in the parking lot, and I saw Jane, the family therapist, kind of – making out – with the guy who usually picks up that little girl – you know, the little blonde girl who always has a violin case. Look, I'll be honest, I don't know if they were making out, but they were awfully close for a really long time. It gave me a funny feeling, and I remembered what you told me about my step-dad, that if I had a wrong feeling, I should tell."
- I'm tired of trying to make you understand. What is so difficult about this? John gets it right away. I guess he's got a little more real-life experience than you do. I bet you just go to your school books and think you can look me up."

Disturbing the equilibrium. These are strategies to make the staff person uncomfortable, off-centered, or uneasy.
- They might say something over the line, and then when confronted, laugh and say they were just joking.
- Manipulators stare, intimidate, and mumble to elicit a negative response, which then justifies their aggression.
- They may make a sudden movement, such as a mock attack, and then smile and say, "Just kidding."

Using the victim's role. Manipulators will often use a victim role – even a real history – as leverage, trying to elicit "privileged guilt."
- "You've never lived our kind of life."
- "I wish I had the kind of chances you had. I probably wouldn't be here today."
- "I was abused by my father . . ." (The most powerful manipulation can be the truth).

A further aspect of this is when the manipulative individual *uses* their genuine victimization as license to hurt others and is aided and abetted by his or her counselor, advocate, or case manager. For example, a victim of systematic domestic violence hits her twelve-year-old son, a very angry and aggressive boy, half way between a cuff and a punch on the shoulder. She is effusively apologetic afterward, and asks for help with her anger issues, attributing it to the fact that the boy was acting exactly like her husband used to, and "I just lost it for a second." Her case manager or nurse minimizes the incident, "reclassifying" it as something below the threshold that would require she report it to the police, thinking that the violence is part of her patient's "victimization," a "post-traumatic stress reaction" that can be mitigated in therapy. In fact, the patient in question is, notwithstanding her own abuse at the hands of someone stronger, a violent abuser of her own children.

Blaming. The more responsibility is theirs, the more they blame others. Sometimes such people will blame or attack, and then when confronted, will straight-facedly deny it OR ask a question like, "How come you are so sensitive?"

Bitter complaining. If manipulators don't get what they want, they may complain bitterly how they trusted the counselor and "this is what happens."

Examples: Complaints for advantage
- "I thought you were different."
- "Honestly, when I came here, I didn't expect much anyway. Men have always treated me badly. That's why it hurts so much. I'd come to think you weren't like other guys."
- "I can't believe I told you about my father . . ."

Flirtation. If you do not address flirtation and come-ons right away, it is viewed as implicit acceptance. You are now open to blackmail, and/or at minimum, an escalation of such approaches. Some manipulators will try to flirt with you in front of other people, in a group session, for example, leading others to believe that something *is* going on, that you are too weak to make it stop, or that the manipulative person has special privileges.

Using manipulative language. This can include the following (in addition to the actions described above):

- Denying direct responsibility ("I got caught up in something.")
- Denying personal responsibility ("Nobody told me.")
- Minimizing ("I made a mistake.")
- Colluding while excluding ("You know what I mean." *Or you would, if you were hip*.)
- Obsequious noncompliance ("I don't know.") This is said so the wise counselor will explain to them what they already knew, thereby enabling them to control the staff person because they are speaking at their beck and call.
- Defining something as true, so it now must be true ("Honestly," or "I'll tell you the truth," or "I wouldn't lie to you.")
- You are like all the rest ("I should have known you wouldn't understand.")

CHAPTER 13

A Wolf in Sheep's Clothing:
The Danger of Psychopathic Individuals
in a Hospital Setting

Highlighting the Psychopath

Everything I have just discussed regarding manipulative strategies (Chapter 12) and will discuss concerning rage (Section IX) is relevant in a discussion of psychopathic individuals. Here, I will discuss the subject of maintaining a safe milieu and, in particular, the safety of your patients, when a psychopathic individual is also a patient in your facility. Because of the extreme risk these relatively rare (an estimated 1 to 3 percent of the population) individuals present, I've included this stand-alone chapter for easy reference.

The terms psychopath and sociopath[4] – you can consider them as interchangeable – evoke very strong reactions in most people. The entertainment media as well as sensationalized news accounts of horrendously violent killers and rapists have introduced into the public's consciousness an image of the malevolent criminal mastermind or the sadistic murdering predator. Violent psychopaths do exist, but they are often rather mundane in appearance and affect, blending in with their surroundings without attracting much attention. Instead of some movie monster such as Hannibal Lector, a much more useful image would be Johnny Depp's character in *Pirates of the Caribbean*. In his role as Captain Jack Sparrow, Depp plays an aggressive narcissist; he is not only charming and likeable but also extremely self-involved and selfish, and quite willing to violate social norms. The only thing he truly cares about is himself. A second image would be the Matt Damon character in *The Talented Mr. Ripley*, an inoffensive chameleon-like man who has no desire to kill anyone, but when circumstances "require" it, he does so without hesitation.

Psychopathic individuals can be disarming in their presentation and show real creativity. They are often very charming and ingratiate themselves to others. The manipulative strategies discussed in Chapter 12 are relevant to understanding the psychopath. However, the psychopathic person presents problems beyond what you will experience with either the "ordinary" criminal personality, or the person with another personality disorder, no matter how disturbed and disturbing they may be.

Just as nature's predators live on the most vulnerable members of the herd, the psychopath preys on the most vulnerable members of society. Therefore, the psychopath will gravitate to your most vulnerable patients. They study everyone with whom they come into contact, making note of any apparent weaknesses, which they then use to their advantage. Not only do they lack a sense of remorse at the harm inflicted upon their victims, but they also often take uncommon delight in such destruction. Such people view the use of a rumor or provocations that evoke an unprofessional response that damages or destroys a staff person's career as a marvelous victory.

Due to their grandiose narcissism, they do not view themselves as being in your program to change their character or actions. Every time they con a professional, their grandiosity increases, leading them to feel a sense of being invulnerable. There are NO therapeutic interventions that can "cure" the psychopathic personality. They actually study mental health professionals' therapeutic interventions as new methods to manipulate others. For example, a psychopath might think, "Wow, when Ms. Gibbs tilts her head and smiles while I'm talking, I find myself relaxing a little. I can use this the next time I'm trying to get close to a child."

Without a doubt, the most dangerous are the sexually violent psychopaths. They groom vulnerable patients for exploitation, or even worse, enact sexual assaults, or on a more mundane level, have sex with whomever they can, simply to gratify a need, heedless of the chaos they create. Although common sense would cause my reader to assume that no hospital or mental health professional would ever engage in a personal relationship with such an individual, a psychopathic individual may attempt to groom and seduce their therapist, physician, or case manager, either for the thrill of destroying their career, or for the purposes of blackmail or privilege. Surprisingly frequently, they are successful. One irony is that it is the most dangerous patients who are most likely to succeed in fostering such a relationship. Metaphorically speaking, ask yourself: Is there anything more beautiful than a leopard?

Many psychopaths are violent:
- Some exhibit an explosive violence. They may lash out with appalling hatred and rage if they are frustrated in their desires or proven out in some way so they feel exposed.
- Some exhibit expedient, predatory aggression. These individuals see it as either a business or a nourishment problem. There is simply something they want and violence is the means to get it.
- Some exhibit sadistic violence. The act of violence itself is gratifying.

Not all psychopaths are "apex predators," like tigers or sharks. Many are fundamentally parasitic. They may spend their time manipulating or stealing possessions from other patients. They may set up others to create emotional drama or conflict, using both patients and staff as toys – "human yo-yos" to dangle on a psychological string. Words are tools to them – thus, the truth and a lie have exactly the same valence, because the only thing that matters is their words' effect on others.

Many psychopaths are impulsive. Their grandiosity often leads them to ignore consequences. Imagine jumping off a cliff to experience the fall without any concern about what might happen at the bottom.

Such individuals owe their allegiance to no one, although they may form quasi-sentimental attachments that last until a stronger interest or desire pushes it away. This loyalty is on the level of, "Who do you think you are, patting my dog without my permission?"

Beyond all else, their highest goal is conning, demeaning, manipulating, and even destroying other people. Helping professionals are particularly attractive targets. Members of your hospital staff are manipulated for the fun of it and studied for useful techniques. They are objects of wrath, at times, and targets for the alleviation of boredom. It is a marvelous victory for such a person to seduce a nurse, counselor, or other member of your staff, thereby ruining his or her career. The destruction of a vulnerable human being is far more delightful than the sex.

Even more important, psychopaths can be devastating to other patients. They undermine group therapy or meetings, setting one person against another. They will play patients against each other so that their conflict allows the psychopath to continue his or her depredations undetected. On other occasions, they will set up other patients, spreading rumors or telling lies so that the more vulnerable or sensitive get in arguments or fights that they can watch for their own amusement. As described above, some will exploit or savagely abuse others the way a fox left in a henhouse will kill all the hens, the walls making it impossible for any of them to escape.

Risks Presented by the Psychopathic Patient

You will be attacked through your best <u>and</u> your worst points. It seems quite logical that the psychopathic individual will attack your weak points – and they certainly do. If you are insecure about your personal appearance, for example, the psychopath will either make you feel more insecure, or in a more sophisticated tactic, reassure you that he or she, at least, finds you quite attractive. What is harder to notice is when you are attacked through your best points. For example, if you are religious, they will consult with you about part of the Bible or the Koran that they do not understand. If you love children, they will find a way to ask your advice on an alleged phone call from their paramour about putting their child on medications. They might really have a child who needs medication! But they are asking you to gain some traction, not to get your help. For such an individual, anything can be leverage. Remember, they don't even have to lie. The truth is an even better tool.

Particularly with forensic patients, listen carefully and verify if what they say is true. Address the problem at face value, but stay absolutely mindful if the patient makes any move to "bond" with you regarding your response. You certainly can answer a question about the Bible or medications or any other issue, if it is something you know about and if it doesn't interfere with either your responsibilities or the treatment plan. Simply remain aware if in doing so you begin to let your guard down.

Notice when WE find ourselves making excuses by "contextualizing" what they are doing. When conned or manipulated, we often find a way to rationalize what the psychopath is doing or has done. For example, after an assault, a staff person says, "You have to understand. He was brought up that way. When Dr. Samuelson ordered him back to his room, it was like a flashback to the way his father treated him."

You may be intimidated. The most obvious manifestation of intimidation is fear. If you are frightened of a patient, immediately consult with other staff and supervisors. <u>Fear always has a reason</u>. What is more difficult to perceive is when we unconsciously avoid being frightened by colluding or giving in to the psychopath. Ironically, the intimidated person may sometimes claim that they have a special rapport or working relationship with the aggressor. In fact, all they are doing is giving the predatory individual what he or she wants.

Be aware of grooming behaviors. The grooming cycle is a pattern of behavior designed to alleviate the intended victim's fears and apprehensions, all the while targeting them for attack. The predatory individual will make their target feel a little off-balance, making them anxious, scared, or flattered. Then they lessen the pressure *while making a request that the staff person would have granted anyway.* Grooming tactics can include momentary trespass on the staff person's personal space or hard eye contact. Just as you start to become uncomfortable, the psychopathic individual moves back a little, or softens or breaks the eye contact, *coupled with a request that you would have granted anyway, such as, "Can I have a glass of water?"* The psychopathic individual begins to "train" the staff person so that, bit-by-bit, they feel reassured, even comfortable, in granting requests to the patient. Eventually, they will ask you to do something just barely "over the line." Once you have crossed a moral or ethical boundary, you are vulnerable to being blackmailed, each time with the promise of release if you do this "one thing." By controlling the victim's emotions, the psychopathic individual is able to maneuver and manipulate that individual into a compromising position, where they may be attacked.

Guard all personal information. As discussed previously, personal information can be used in a variety of ways, and the psychopath can use such information to determine points of leverage against you. They can talk publicly about you, apparently displaying intimate knowledge of your affairs. In the worst case, such information can be used to track you down outside of your professional life, or make you fear for the safety of your friends and family.

Do not get beyond the horizon line. <u>Do not meet psychopaths alone!</u> You are vulnerable to false accusations; with no one to monitor the interaction, you are vulnerable to manipulation that you may not even perceive happening; and of course, you are vulnerable to attack.

Calculated splitting. As stated earlier, the psychopathic individual uses gossip, rumors, misdirection, and blatant lying to set all the stakeholders involved in their supervision and treatment against each other. Regular communication and consultation with the various members of the treatment team is the best way to detect and confront calculated splitting and rumor-mongering.

Do not try to "out-tough" the psychopath. There are, I believe, two types of psychopaths: those who live as if they have nothing to lose, and those who *believe* that they live this way. In either case, such individuals are exquisitely skilled in reading other people: how strong they are, what limits beyond which their target cannot be pushed, and, what danger they can present. Those of us who have a lot to lose – our reputations, our careers, and our well-being – cannot successfully "bring off" an appearance of being a "pirate" ourselves. This does not mean we cannot prevail in an interaction with a predatory individual. We can! The best protection against psychopathic manipulation is control of oneself, both centering and being aware of one's strengths and vulnerabilities (Section IV). Rather than trying to appear tough, we must be people of integrity. The more we hew to the highest professional standards and the more comfortable we are in our own skins, the less vulnerable we are to psychopathic manipulation.

What to Do When a Patient Exhibits Psychopathic Behaviors

You must become familiar with the behaviors of such individuals. I strongly recommend Robert Hare's *Without Conscience: The Disturbing World of the Psychopath*.[5] In agencies that may have a number of such patients, such as forensic units or mental health wards in jails or prisons, it would prove very valuable that you send at least one person to become certified in Hare's assessment procedures.[6]

Consult and consult again. Do not discount the observations of line staff, or sometimes surprisingly important, support and custodial staff, who interact most directly with the patient. Consult yet again. Discuss splitting, which, for the psychopath, is a conscious process. Unlike the unconscious splitting of the borderline personality, it is used to engender conflict or amusement.

Recognize that the patient whom you consider your star, the one to whom you devote the most energy or attention, may in fact have successfully groomed you. Therefore, do not only consult about those who disquiet you. Consult about those with whom you believe you are doing your best work.

Inpatient psychiatrists must diagnose psychopathy when they see it, even if that is not the diagnosis of the outpatient treatment provider. I have observed, all too often, inpatient psychiatrists who allow a misguided "professional courtesy" to trump good practice. If a psychiatrist does not properly diagnose such individuals, but instead maintains an outpatient practitioner's diagnosis of, for example, bipolar disorder that is either incorrect or incomplete, that doctor runs the risk of being culpable for any harm that results to patients and staff. The diagnosing psychiatrist must follow up with outpatient treatment providers and clearly explain why he or she has settled on the psychopathic diagnosis and what the implications are for both inpatient and outpatient treatment.

If you are a forensic hospital, you very likely will have psychopathic patients. You must develop policies on how best to manage such individuals, including implementing sanctions for the behaviors they will surely enact and creating a strong, comprehensive plan to protect more vulnerable patients.

Once you realize that a person is primarily psychopathic, you must accept that you will not be able to cure them. A basic formula is "monitor, not therapy." If there are medical issues to address, then, by all means, do so. If the patient needs further psychiatric assessment, this, too, should be done. Beyond this, your task is the protection of both patients and staff. All staff must be alerted to the individual's style of aggression and/or manipulation, and every staff meeting must include an update on the patient's behaviors.

If you are an ordinary, rather than forensic psychiatric hospital, you must strive to discharge such individuals as quickly as you can. For someone to be in a psychiatric hospital, there must be both a treatment plan and a treatment goal. Once you realize that they are primarily psychopathic, your treatment goal must be protection of your patients and staff. The same is true for many residential treatment facilities and group homes.

If you are a substance abuse treatment facility, you have a particular problem. Many substance abusers act in sociopathic ways while in the throes of their addiction. Therefore, you must maintain adequate training in recognizing such behaviors, whether substance/lifestyle induced or innate. Beyond this, you must learn to cut your losses. <u>People with addiction issues in remission who are truly engaged in treatment usually begin to abandon manipulative and strategic behaviors. True psychopaths, on the other hand, do not</u>. They may use different strategies when they are sober, but they will never abandon a tactical, manipulative approach. If you see no improvement, or worse, an increase in chaos in the milieu associated with their presence, staff must ask if the patient is psychopathic. If you do not expel such individuals, they will jeopardize the sobriety of all your other patients.

Psychopathic individuals are, by nature, profoundly dangerous to everyone, both on a physical and psychological level. <u>Staff and patients will be at risk as long as the psychopath is enrolled in your services</u>. You have a moral responsibility to protect your patients and fellow staff – and beyond that, who wants to have their own life destroyed by someone you are trying to help? Therefore, learn to recognize the psychopath, that 1 to 3 percent or so of the population who swims through people like a shark through a school of fish, focused on no other needs than his or her own. Furthermore, get them out of your hospital as quickly as possible <u>unless you can define and document cogent clinical reasons that they should stay, along with an ironclad plan to keep everyone safe in the process</u>. Consider, for example, a woman with both bipolar disorder and psychopathic personality. She has a treatable condition, as far as her bipolar disorder is concerned, one that probably makes her antisocial behavior worse. She needs help. This will not be easy, however. To use a crude metaphor, imagine her as a jaguar with a thorn in her paw. She is in terrible pain. She needs help. You cannot, however, simply offer your lap and your hands to cradle those terrible talons, while you dig into her flesh to pull out the thorn. You must be safe to help.

SECTION III

Communication with Those with Severe Mental Illness or Other Conditions that Cause Severe Disability

CHAPTER 14

Struggling in a Fog:
Dealing with Symptoms
of Disorganization

What is Disorganization?

Disorganization is a general term to describe what it is like when individuals cannot adequately organize their cognitions, perceptions, and/or feelings so that they can function well in the real world. Please note that, as elsewhere in this book, I am referring to behavioral manifestations, not the inner experience of the disorganized person, because, as you will see below, I include quite different types of individuals within the disorganized rubric.

Among the many causes of disorganization and delirium are metabolic or infectious disorders. For this reason, severe disorganization should always be regarded, first and foremost, as a medical emergency until such causes have been ruled out. If not immediately attended to, such disorders can cause permanent, even life-threatening, damage.

Disorganized people may, perhaps, be *autistic*, overwhelmed by the incomprehensible emotional communications of people, as well as the overly rich and complex sensory impressions that they receive. When colors have sounds, and music creates odors and swathes of light, autistic individuals may become rapt or lost in the experience. Of all that is in the world, however, the most incomprehensible to the autistic person is interaction with other human beings.

Developmentally delayed individuals often lack the maturity to manage complex or frustrating situations. In addition, due to their cognitive limitations, they are not skilled at problem-solving situations.

Profoundly psychotic people (Chapters 17 and 18) also become disorganized. When one becomes disorganized, even one's delusions break down into chaos. Oddly enough, delusions, despite the myriad problems they cause, are an organizing principle. If you believe yourself to be surrounded by enemies or on a mission to save the world, you have concentration and a somewhat coherent idea of what to do next, delusional though it may be.

Severe intoxication, withdrawal from and long-term damage from intoxicating substances, creates disorganized, even delirious states.

All of these problems can also apply to someone who is demented due to head injury, Alzheimer's disease, or other forms of senility. Finally, severely traumatized individuals can become so overwhelmed that they shift into a chaotic, disorganized state.

The near impossibility of communication

You will know you are dealing with a disorganized person because they are nearly incoherent, or it is otherwise impossible to communicate with them. They may seem to shift from one emotion to another, for no logical reason, and it is very hard, if not impossible, to hold their attention.

Small Bits at a Time

To better communicate with disorganized patients, divide tasks and instructions into small bits. For example, it is unreasonable to expect disorganized individuals, unattended, to do something as complex as cleaning up their room, which can include picking up, folding, and putting away clothes; making the bed; and other tasks. The texture of the towel they are folding, for example, or the play of light on the floor may distract some disorganized people. Others get confused and aimlessly move things around. Make sure that you are very specific when you give instructions. There is no point in being irritable. That just makes things harder for these individuals because they usually do not know why you are upset. This becomes an added disorganizing factor.

Not only should your instructions be specific, but they should also be simple and divided in small manageable bits. Your sentences should be short. Each sentence should have only one important message, and it is likely that even in the best of circumstances, you will have to repeat this message several times before it sinks in. Rather than saying, "Pick up your clothes," you may have to say, "Pick up your red shirt. Put it on the bed. Pick up your plaid dress. Put that on the bed too. Fold your red shirt." If you really want your disorganized patient to accomplish a task, you may have to firmly but kindly supervise them every step of the way.

Of course, you should hold your patient to a high standard: just don't make it an impossible one.

Let Me Repeat Myself

When we are not understood, our usual impulse is to elaborate: we use different words and expressive hand and facial gestures, and we intensify the emotional tone of our communication. With disorganized people, it is often better to simply repeat the same statement or question word-for-word, sometimes four, five or more times. Repetition becomes a touchstone of stability. It is the one consistent point at that

DEALING WITH SYMPTOMS OF DISORGANIZATION

moment. The aim is not to browbeat them. You should not increase your volume, shouting at them to get through to them. If you change your vocal tone or get irritated, you will absolutely defeat the purpose of repetition. If you keep your nonverbal communication stable and calm, the disorganized individual will become more, rather than less, under control.

> **Examples: Here is an example of first the wrong way, and then the right way to communicate with a disorganized patient in an assisted living situation:**
>
> "You've left your chores long enough. This room is a mess, and you've just put it off too long. Now there is mold on the carpet, and it smells terrible. I don't know where we can even begin. This place is horrible!"
>
> *Rather than venting your feelings toward him, your tone of voice should be firm, calm, and with little emotion other than, possibly, some warmth.*
> - Jiro, it is time to do your chores.
> - Put down the book, Jiro. Jiro, put down the book. Jiro, put down the book. *(This is not done in a nagging tone. The three sentences are said slowly, with pauses between them, to give Jiro time to act).*
> - Good. Stand up.
> - Stand up, Jiro. Good.
> - Pick up your clothes and put them on the bed.
> - Pick up your clothes and put them on the bed.
>
> Imagine that this is too "big" a task. He seems overwhelmed. So you re-adjust:
> - Jiro, pick up the red sweater and put it on the bed. Good.
> - Jiro, pick up the blue jeans and put them on the bed.
>
> It may make you uncomfortable to be so direct. Naturally, you will have to figure out a style that works best for you and your patient. "Please" might be a good idea, or it may not. Remember that "please" and "thank you" are added information, and <u>with a really concrete or disorganized individual, more information does not help.</u> It is far kinder to be clear than to be polite.

Creating Room for Success

Your patient should have daily tasks that are necessary, but are also failure-free. Life should not be a perpetual struggle – one needs to be successful at something, no matter how small. While positive reinforcement is usually rewarding to anyone, it can mean a great deal to mentally ill and disorganized individuals. Indeed, for some people, this may be the only positive feedback they have ever received, and it will often help them focus on their treatment issues.

Behavioral Charts

Behavioral charts can be very helpful for some people. First of all, tasks are divided into small bits. You also have a check-off chart where everyone can see what has to be done and how much has been accomplished.

Be Aware of and Attend to Sensory Needs

Loud noises may be distracting or overwhelming. Lights may be too bright and glaring. The music you play may be irritating or disturbing. Consider what kind of environment would make your patients feel most comfortable, safe, and stable. Although there is certainly a limit on how closely you can approach this ideal, your working relationship with your patients will be much more positive if the environment is one in which they feel comfortable.

Magical Thinking

This is a term that overlaps with delusions (Chapter 17). Magical thinking is telling stories that one then believes. It is most common among small children, senile and demented adults, and developmentally delayed individuals. Unlike psychotic delusions, magical thinking does not have the same enclosed quality, where a fundamental truth is revealed suddenly and then locked into place in the person's mind. Rather, what arises within the disorganized person's mind and fantasies is repeated, proclaimed, and then believed.

Magical thinking sometimes emerges out of a confused state, where the mind latches on to a detail of what is perceived and constructs a story around it. John, for example, notices that he and his case manager are both physically round and wear glasses, so he honestly believes that his case manager is his grandmother. In other cases, it can also be fable making – the kinds of stories very young people tell.

Example: Magical thinking

A developmentally disabled teenager, with a long history of aggression, confided to me that he could heal knife wounds. "You just peel off the skin of a salmon and put it over the wound. It'll be totally healed in one night. There won't even be a scar."

Once you've established that a claim or statement is not true, there is little to be gained by arguing with the patient about magical thinking. Sometimes, just let it go. Other times, you can say, even with a little tiredness in your voice, "I've heard that story before. You don't have to tell me again." Or, "Let's not talk about that anymore. What do you want to have for dinner tonight?" Then, simply move on to the next topic at hand and shift the patient's focus toward issues of immediate concern.

Review: Dealing with symptoms of disorganization

You will know you are dealing with a disorganized patient when you notice the following:

- The patient is nearly incoherent, and it may be nearly impossible to communicate with them.
- The patient seems to shift from one emotion to another, with no logical reason or explanation.
- Focusing their attention is very hard, if not impossible.
- They may offer statements – magical thinking – that, unlike delusions, have the naïve character of a child's fantasies.

Remember:

- Divide tasks into small bits.
- Give simple, specific instructions.
- Be realistic about what the patient can and cannot do.
- Repeat your instructions rather than elaborate on them. Do not change your vocal tone.
- Do not argue with magical thinking; redirect the patient to the task and issues at hand.

CHAPTER 15

Dropping Stones in a Well:
Latency

What is latency?

You will recognize latency when the person to whom you are speaking not only delays his or her answers but also replies with somewhat odd and disjointed answers that aren't related to your questions. This is different from being silent or defying you. You get the sense that they are not "there" – that it is about something going on inside of them, and not about you at all.

Latency is a behavior that is often a manifestation of disorganization, but because of both its significance and its confusing nature, it is productive to discuss it as an entity of its own. This is a behavior in which people respond to communication in a very slow manner. You might ask a question and they quietly talk to themselves as they puzzle out what you might be saying, or they may engage in odd stereotypical movements, which might either have a meaning important only to them or may be a self-soothing behavior. Some latent individuals may simply stare away with a vacuous look on their face.

Some people who are manifesting latency may be very confused: you might say, "Take care," meaning, "Good-bye, I hope all goes well for you," and they, being very concrete (Chapter 1), wonder, "Take care of what?" Others may be hearing voices inside their head or be overwhelmed by stimuli from outside – the glitter of light on the varnish of the piano and the white keys that look like teeth – and your words seem very far away. Others may be very cognitively impaired and they simply do not understand what you are saying.

Were you to drop a stone in a well, you would expect to hear a splash as the stone hits the water at the bottom. This is the experience of communicating with a healthy person: what you say "hits bottom." Imagine the latent mind like a very old well, with bricks sticking out and a tangle of tree roots halfway down. The stone hits the roots and bounces off a brick, then another and another. This time, you don't hear a splash – you hear nothing. So you start throwing more stones, one after another. You now have any number of stones bouncing around, colliding into each other, adding to your frustration and their confusion, without the first stone ever reaching the bottom of the well. In other words, adding more words doesn't enhance communication with latent individuals.

Coping with Latency: Keep Things Simple

Be patient. Although communicating with such a patient can be frustrating and often time consuming, you must remain calm if you hope to succeed in communicating with the latent individual. Indeed, any frustration or anger you display will only further confuse the patient.

Keep your sentences and instructions short and direct. Minimize all the qualifiers – such as "you might," "maybe," and "kind of" – that you ordinarily put in your sentences.

Don't dance when you talk. Try to minimize your changeable hand gestures and facial expressions. This does not mean you should speak robotically, but simplicity is best.

Repeat. Latent people usually do **not** need things explained in further detail; they just didn't get it the first time. So, say the same thing again. <u>Make sure you use the same tone of voice when your repeat yourself. Adding other emotions is overloading the communication with new data that they have to try to understand.</u> Repetition is like somehow throwing the *same* pebble down the well, reinforcing the original. Rather than adding a new stone, you've added weight to the one already there. It has, metaphorically speaking, "double mass." Now the stone can get through the roots and bricks and hit bottom.

Repeat back. When you think your communication has been successful, try to get the patient to repeat the instructions back to you in their own words.

Communication with the latent patient
- Be patient.
- Keep your sentences short and direct.
- Minimize hand gestures and changeable facial expressions.
- Repeat the instructions, using the same words and the same tone of voice.
- Try to get the latent individual to repeat back your instructions.

CHAPTER 16

Withdrawal from
Intoxicating Substances

First and foremost, alcohol and drug withdrawals are medical emergencies. Therefore, if *your* patient is in withdrawal, they are in the right place. They are either in the hospital or detox center being treated for this medical emergency; or if they are in an evaluation and treatment unit of a mental health agency, they have been medically cleared (the withdrawal symptoms are at a stage that does not pose a substantial medical risk). If a person in the latter setting starts to display symptoms of withdrawal, it has *become* a medical emergency, and they must be either treated on the spot or taken to an emergency unit of a hospital.

People in withdrawal are often in pain or feeling quite ill. They may also be frightened or irritable and very much focused, in a completely self-centered way, on getting their needs met. Paradoxically, they may display a high level of resistance to accepting proper medical attention, or insist that they are well enough to be left alone. You will often be quite familiar with these individuals because of their prior history with your hospital. Not infrequently, you have even seen them recently intoxicated. The signs of withdrawal (and proper response) can include the following:
- Unstable coordination. Try to get them to sit or lie down for their safety.
- Restlessness and agitation. Try to reduce any stimulating input.
- Unpredictable and sudden actions. Keep your movements calm and slow so that you do not elicit their startle reflex, which can easily turn into an attack.
- Slurred or incoherent speech. Speak in a calm, quiet voice and make an extra effort to understand what they are saying. Provide short explanations.
- Abnormally rigid muscles.
- Being argumentative and demanding. Try to redirect or de-escalate them depending on the mode of anger or rage they exhibit.

Calming Individuals in Withdrawal
Be calm and firm. Redirect them when they get very demanding, and reassure them that help is on the way. To reiterate, this is a medical emergency. You are simply trying to calm them until the necessary help arrives, or the palliative treatments you have initiated take effect.

For the purposes of de-escalation, there is no specific state of withdrawal anger or rage. The individual in withdrawal, if enraged, will shift into one of the modes of anger or rage outlined in the latter sections of this book. You will, therefore, control and de-escalate them based on what mode of rage that they are exhibiting.

The question of dual diagnosis

Given all the attention paid to this subject, the reader may question why there is not a large section devoted to the behaviors of "dual-diagnosis" patients (those with both substance abuse and mental health issues) as a separate concern. There is no doubt, whatsoever, that dual diagnosis can profoundly affect every aspect of an individual's life. Substance abuse makes it much harder to heal from or even manage mental illness, and mental illness makes it much harder to recover from substance abuse.

This book, however, is concerned with the issues of safety and de-escalation of those in extreme states. Imagine all the descriptions of behavior necessary to distinguish between, for example, a solvent-inhaling person with bipolar disorder, a marijuana-smoking person with social phobia, and a schizophrenic who injects a mixture of cocaine and heroin. Other patients may be experiencing severe reactions brought on by mixing drugs or alcohol with their prescribed psychotropic medications. To be sure, each and all of these concerns are relevant when it comes to treatment and finding resources to best help the patient. The only thing that we are focusing on, however, is behavior. Whatever substances they may have ingested, whatever illness or syndrome they may be suffering from, we are concerned with the behaviors that they are displaying. This is the only data relevant for crisis intervention. In a crisis, deal with the behavior, not the cause.

CHAPTER 17

Psychosis: Delusions and Hallucinations

> **Psychosis: A complex of behaviors, not a diagnosis**
>
> Whatever the diagnosis, be it schizophrenia, bipolar disorder, depression, trauma induced, or drug provoked, psychosis is typified by delusions and/or hallucinations. This is NOT a comprehensive clinical definition; however, the term "psychosis" is used in this book to denote a complex of behaviors that appears in people with a variety of diagnoses and demands a particular set of responses.

What is a Delusion?

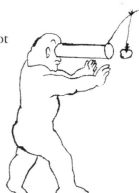

A *delusion* is first and foremost a disturbance in cognition, a belief that does not fit reality. What this means is not as simple as it sounds.

- People from different cultures have different beliefs. Shared cultural beliefs, however, are not delusional, even if you cannot conceive how other people could see the world as they do.
- Sometimes, there is nothing remarkable about the delusional belief, except that it is not true. For example, everyone knows the FBI follows people; the question in this case becomes, "Is the FBI following this particular patient?"
- A lot of people have eccentric ideas: unconventional religious beliefs; nontraditional dietary and health habits; a belief in aliens, crop circles, or telepathy. Possibly, some of these are *your* beliefs; they are eccentric to me, but not to you. Perhaps some of mine are eccentric to you. However, unique or unusual ideas and beliefs are not delusional.

Delusions are like cults with one member. When people become delusional, it is as if they have had a revelation. Suddenly, the truth comes to them. All the confusing thoughts they have had, all the worries, prayers, fantasies, or ideas suddenly coalesce into the **BELIEF**. Such beliefs are unshakable, unarguable, and unalterable by conflicting evidence.

Types of Delusions

Grandiose delusions. People believe that they have been appointed on a special mission, possess extraordinary or unusual powers, or are special, remarkable beings.

Religious delusions. Often linked with grandiose delusions, such patients may become preoccupied with religion, focusing all their attention on their beliefs, which may be self-made or associated with mainstream doctrines.

Jealous delusions. The patient may believe, against all evidence, that their partner is unfaithful to them. Many people experience jealousy, and are often quite irrational. Jealous delusions, however, are far different from illogical or insecure emotions. The jealous delusional patient concocts infidelity out of the slightest glance, a change in clothing, or a five-minute delay in returning home. Male perpetrators of domestic violence, particularly those with a paranoid or borderline character structure (Chapters 10 and 11) often manifest this type of delusional psychosis in periods of stress.

Delusional stalking.[7] People believe that another person is in love with them, is married to them, or has somehow been designated as theirs, whether they know it or not. Delusional stalking is termed erotomania.

Persecutory delusions (paranoia). Such people may believe that they have enemies: People, institutions, or other powers have hostile intentions toward them, or may be committing evil actions against them. The paranoid individual is a grandiose victim. Such individuals often have "ideas of reference." They believe that others are sending energy toward them, thinking about them, talking about them, or looking at them with malevolent intent. The paranoid character has already been discussed (Chapter 10). Delusional paranoia is far more than a mere attitude. It is an unshakable belief, bolstered by perceptions (hallucinations and false interpretations of others' actions).

What are Hallucinations?

A *hallucination* is a disturbance in perception. One perceives things in a way that does not conform to reality. Hallucinations are often, but not always, accompanied by delusions.

One can hallucinate without being psychotic

It is possible to perceive a hallucination without being delusional or psychotic. For example, after several days of jet lag, some people complain of hearing voices, something they usually describe as quite unpleasant. However, they are quite aware that the voices are caused by sleep-deprivation and pay them no more heed than people do when they have a song – usually trite or banal, like an advertisement jingle – stuck in their head.

Types of Hallucinations

One can experience hallucinations with any of one of the senses:

Auditory hallucinations. There are two levels of auditory hallucinations. The first level is **auditory distortion**. One mishears what is said. For example, a person experiencing paranoia is in the middle of a restaurant and they hear someone say, "Say, do you want the chicken or the ribs?" They hear, "Let's say we get this chicken in the ribs." People with persecutory delusions often display a "listening attitude." They enter a situation that evokes their paranoia and expect to be victimized, accused, talked about, or assaulted. They either mishear people based on what they expect to hear, or in more severe cases, they truly hear hallucinatory voices uttering just what they expected or feared.[88]

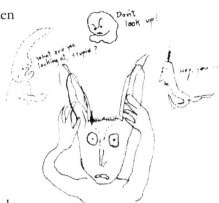

The second level is true **auditory hallucinations**. Close your eyes when someone speaks to you. Do you still hear their voice? When people have an auditory hallucination, it is that real. It is not imagination – it is an experience. That is why you cannot simply say, "The voice isn't real." That makes as much sense to them as someone telling you that the lightening and thunder that just shorted out your electricity and then shook your house didn't happen.

The Torment of Hallucinations

Hallucinations torment their victims in a variety of ways:

- For unknown reasons, hallucinated voices are almost always cruel. People can be ordered to do awful or degrading things, or they may simply hear awful sounds and ugly demeaning words. Visual hallucinations can be as haunting as ghosts. Olfactory hallucinations are often foul odors, and tactile hallucinations are almost always very unpleasant sensations.
- People try to tell others what they perceive, but their experience is denied over and over again. They can be teased or laughed at. Ironically, the people they tell often torment them in ways similar to the torment of the hallucinations.

Psychotic people find that their worldview is called into question every day. They don't know what is real and what is not. Imagine reaching to pick up your tea, and not knowing if the liquid will disappear, or if the handle of the cup will suddenly twine around your finger like a little snake. Imagine this is true of every object in your life. In such circumstances, the person finds it difficult to trust anything at all.

Hallucinations can be horrible

I have interviewed people who have watched their bodies rotting, seen people on the street turn into deformed monsters, and wounds open up on their bodies. Beasts emerge from wall hangings, and satanic claws edge around a doorframe. All too often, the hallucinations are nightmarish.

Hallucinations are not *necessarily* horrible

Some people have hallucinations that function like guardian angels, cautioning them how to act. Sometimes this is actually helpful, whereas at other times, the voices, although ostensibly benign, encourage the person toward actions that cause them problems.

CHAPTER 18

Communication with Someone
Who Is Experiencing Delusions
or Hallucinations

Paraphrasing for psychotic individuals

Aside from the specific communication strategies in this chapter, a wonderful method of communication with all people in heightened states of stress, and particularly useful with psychotic individuals, is paraphrasing (Chapter 44).

Disengage

Communicating with a psychotic person can be very draining, even maddening. Like a cultist trying to convert you to their group, the patient may try to convince you that what they believe is real. They may insist that you accept their beliefs, or even more problematic, insist that you *do* believe but simply won't admit it. If you try to argue with them, they may become more focused on debating your resistance or furious that you deny what is, to them, absolutely true.

There is often no good reason to continue such a discussion. Delusions are not like some sort of backed-up fluid that you vent and drain away. While delusional people may feel locked in their own inner world and desperate to communicate what they are experiencing, discussion and argument seem to cement the delusions even further – the more one talks about it, the more one believes it to be true and, often, more excited and agitated as well.

Rule #1: Disengage

There are many occasions when nothing at all can be accomplished by talking about delusions or hallucinations. In such cases, disengage, especially if further discussion tends to elicit an angry or irrational response from the patient.

Islands of Sanity

Imagine being dropped overboard into the ocean, with its cold and buffeting waves, not to mention everything from sharks to jellyfish. This is like the delusional world: it is so overwhelming that it seems inescapable. Even in the ocean, however, there are small patches of land – islands. If you can only get to them, you can put your feet on solid ground.

For the psychotic individual, there are "islands of sanity," areas of their lives where they are not delusional. They may be convinced, for example, that someone is poisoning their food and only canned goods are safe to eat, or that someone is beaming messages directly into their brain. Imagine, however, that you begin talking about football, and as you begin discussing the Pittsburgh Steelers' next game, the patient, without even realizing it, takes their mind off their delusions. They have a moment of respite. If you steer conversations toward these islands of sanity, they may begin to associate you with a sense of stability, someone with whom they can have moments of clarity and peace.

Rule #2: Move toward the islands of sanity

Pay attention to areas of thought and subjects where your patient is not delusional, and talk about those subjects whenever possible. Link one island of sanity with other islands – think of yourself as expanding the size of the landmass, creating an area where life is predictable and safe. If the patient gets stuck within his or her delusions, you may find that changing the subject requires real finesse. Nonetheless, do so whenever you can, because talking about the delusion often makes things worse for the patient. Talking about "healthy" subjects brings peace.

When *Should* You Talk about the Delusions?

Some of the people of greatest concern are those you see over and over again. Because they frequently decompensate, or go off their medications, it is necessary to do a brief threat assessment every time you see them.

Let us imagine that your patient is sure that he is the Archangel Michael. If you recall this biblical story, Michael casts Satan out of heaven. Michael is power incarnate, the righteous sword of the Lord God. Further, imagine that your patient sometimes believes he perceives Satan's work in the behavior of people around him. On one occasion, he was arrested after hammering on his neighbor's door, armed with a sword, yelling that he was going to cut Satan out of the hearts of the children to save them for the Lord. Based on this past history of violence, you *should* ask direct questions about his delusions, whenever he begins to talk about God, angels, Satan, or anything else that is connected to these very dangerous thoughts. For instance, you may ask questions like these:
- "John, are you telling me that you think you have seen Satan? Where?"
- "Why do you think that this is Satan's work?"
- "Do you think you should do anything about this?"
- "What do you think you should do?"

If John's answers are bland and not aggressive, you can change the subject at the appropriate time, shifting to an "island of sanity," for example. If, however, his answers sound potentially dangerous, then you must act. For example, you would obviously have a potential crisis were he to say, "Don't call me John! I'm Michael, the Lord's most beloved angel. Satan will have no place on this earth when I take my righteous sword in my strong right arm!"

Rule #3: Talk about the delusions to assess risk

Talk about the delusions as a means of threat assessment. Ask direct questions, particularly in regard to their intention to hurt themselves or others. If they do not bring such subjects up for discussion, but their delusions have been a problem in the past, occasionally bring up the subject yourself, just to see if they have become decompensated again.

Dangerous answers are an alarm call to get help – alerting his doctor, his care team, and in some cases, the police. He may need his medications adjusted or his stay in the hospital extended. But whatever the appropriate response, you must act when he is dangerous again.

Don't Agree – At Least Most of the Time

Although agreement may seem to be the path of least resistance, doing so can present a number of problems. When you agree with delusions and/or hallucinations, you will entrench them even more deeply into the patient's belief system.

Example #1: The danger of agreeing with delusions

Nadia, for example, constantly struggled with her delusions. She had claimed for years that she was impregnated by one of the bailiffs of the superior court, and that the judge had her child taken away. She was, at times, belligerent and demanding about her belief, but in her heart of hearts, she doubted that it was true. One day a treatment aide, tired of hearing about it, said to her, "Nadia, it's true. There is a service called the Guardians of Light. They were worried about your baby's well-being, because you were really young and your dad is so evil. Your baby is safe. He was adopted into a loving home. You don't have to wonder anymore. Everything is all right. I saw the baby before they took it away. I don't know who they were, but they were driving a black car." From that day on, Nadia's beliefs were locked in. She no longer doubted – and when she introduced the subject again and again, she was much more aggressive than before, because no one was doing anything to help, even though she now *knew* it had to be true.

When you agree with delusions or hallucinations, you can be incorporated into the delusional system. Sometimes this can be ostensibly benign, but wearing. All that happens is that the person incessantly wants to talk about the delusions with the only person who seems to share that point of view. <u>It can be much more dangerous, however.</u>

Example #2: The danger of agreeing with delusions

James plays the guitar. He began to believe that he and Joseph, one of the psych techs, who happened to also be a professional musician (he found this out on Facebook), were part of the same band. Joseph, thinking this was benign, began to agree with this delusion, thinking it would build rapport between them. Over a long weekend, when James was transitioning to another medication, he became convinced that Joseph had stolen a song that they had co-written and sold it to a major record label. James heard it on the radio every day, but he had not been paid for it. Calling him a thief, James attacked Joseph with a chair.

Just because one is mentally ill does not mean the person is gullible or stupid.

Example #3: The danger of agreeing with delusions

Alcee began agreeing with Jeremiah's delusions because he was tired of arguing with him, and hoped that by doing so Jeremiah would be satisfied and stop bringing up the subject. Every time Jeremiah mentioned his fears about the Secret Service, who had an office in the same city, Alcee agreed. However, Jeremiah realized that he was being brushed off – that the psych nurse was patronizing him. He was furious and decided that the best way to show Alcee how upset he'd become was to attack the first staff person who came within six feet of him.

Partial exception to the rule: Sometimes the mentally ill patient may incorporate one or more staff persons into their delusions in a positive way. For example, a patient believes he has a secret team of advisors who tell him what to do. He announces that his case manager is on the team, and he therefore decides to listen to what she says and follow her advice. Do not try to "prime the pump" by claiming a positive role in their delusions, or simply accept it if the patient so "appoints" you. Rather, consider this development from all sides. Consult with the entire treatment team. You have to assess if there is any risk that the delusion might become distorted in a dangerous way. If, in your considered judgment, it does make tactical sense, at *most* you accept this information silently. Don't say it aloud. The healthy aspect of the patient' psychology will detect being conned or leveraged, and you will lose any working rapport you have with them.

Rule #4: Don't pretend to believe or agree with the delusions

Partial exception: If the patient has incorporated a staff person into their delusional system in a benign and positive way, consult with the entire treatment team, weighing any possible benefits and risks. In some cases, staff may <u>passively</u> accept what the patient says as it helps them stabilize within the milieu. Do not, however, bring it up yourself or remind the person of their delusional belief (i.e., "Remember how you said Trent is your guardian angel?"). Reassess during staffing discussions to ensure that it continues to be positive for the patient and for the milieu.

Don't Disagree – At Least Most of the Time

Common sense seems to demand that you speak for reality. When people see something that isn't there, shouldn't you tell them so? If they have an irrational belief, why not argue them out of it, or at least diplomatically point out where they are wrong? This is problematic, however, because you are arguing *reality* with someone.

If someone were to come to your office and tell you that the office walls were red when they are pale green, would you believe them, no matter how intensely they argued the point? If you were having a conversation with your daughter, would you believe someone who told you that you were talking to yourself, that there was no one else in the room?

The fundamental problem with arguing with delusional or hallucinating people is that you are telling them that their senses and their brains are lying to them. Telling them that the world as they perceive it is not real will not improve a therapeutic rapport. Individuals experiencing psychosis find everyday life to be very stressful and sometimes quite frightening. It is very important that you have as few arguments as possible within your clinical setting.

Sometimes, however, a delusional patient may ask, or even plead with you, for disagreement because they do not want to believe what their delusions seem to tell them. At other times, a hallucinating person can make a tenuous distinction between real perceptions and hallucinations and will ask you if you think their hallucination is real. In these cases, *when you have been invited*, it is acceptable to state that not only do you not perceive or believe the hallucination or delusion, but you <u>also</u> do not think it is real.

Rule #5: Don't disagree, at least most of the time

Do not engage in arguments about whether the psychotic person's perceptions are real. You can make an exception – in which you state that you do not believe that the delusional belief is correct or that the hallucination is not real *when* the person doubts its reality and requests a "reality check." Even here, do not simply state, "That's not real." Discuss the situation with the patient for at least a few minutes, so you are clear what they are truly concerned about and what they are asking from you.

An Important Exception to the "Don't Disagree" Rule: Erotomania and Stalking

Stalking delusions are dangerous because they involve another person as the victim. In addition, the patient often has an absolutely selfish, entitled sense of their right to approach or harass the victim, either in person or through the use of electronic media, such as text messages, email, or social networking websites. Stalking is a crime. The victim needs to be protected, something that on a legal and moral basis almost always requires you to call police.[9] That aside, unless you are at risk of assault, you must very calmly, but directly, state that it is not true that the victim is destined for, in love with, or otherwise involved with a given person. Do not get into long discussions, much less arguments. Simply state that it is not true. Otherwise, your "conditional" demurrals may be taken as agreement. Even if you believe that further discussion of their delusions will put you at risk, do not "sell-out" the victim by agreeing with the perpetrator in hopes that this will allow you to extricate yourself. Instead, change the subject, leave their presence as quickly as possible, and gather necessary resources (other staff, security, or police) to ensure immediate safety for those in the hospital and more long-range safety for the potential victim.

Rule #6: Disagree! The exception of erotomania

In almost all cases, you must call the police. Always consult with a legal advisor to determine the rules of confidentiality and duty to warn in such situations. Do not agree with or be noncommittal in regards to their delusions. Disengage, if you are in danger. In all other cases, firmly and directly disagree with the person's delusional belief that they are in a relationship with a person or that the person is destined for them.

Differentiation: A Respectful Way to Distinguish between Your World and Theirs

Psychosis can affect every aspect of a person's existence. It is impossible to escape oneself. Just when you think you are at peace, an ugly voice suddenly rises inside your head and accuses you of something obscene, or as you gaze at the leaves outside your window, you see beings beckoning to you to jump from your window. Worse, much of this is something you cannot share or talk about. People simply disbelieve you, or minimize what troubles or preoccupies you, telling you to stop imagining things. Most tragically, even the people you love are tainted by the psychotic experience – people become terrified or enraged toward those who could, otherwise, be perceived as protecting and caring for them. *It is like seeing yourself in a world of distorted mirrors – wherever you look is just a twisted aspect of yourself.*

When we are in a true relationship, we are face-to-face with someone "other." At any moment, that other can offer you something unexpected, something new. Perceiving the other person through delusions, the person becomes "fixed." That person becomes known in the worst way: always as expected.

When your patient voices a delusion or talks about a hallucination, the surest way to make that vital distinction between your world and theirs is to *differentiate*. This word simply means to perceive or express a difference. You should acknowledge the patient's perceptions and beliefs, while also informing them that, although you do not share their perceptions, you are not arguing that theirs are invalid. You are however, attempting to have the patient also become aware that other viewpoints do exist. Here are some examples:

- Alice, I see the table and chairs, the pictures on the wall, and the books on the floor, but there is something you see that I don't. I do not see a vat of boiling oil in the corner of the room. No, I'm not saying you don't see it. I believe you do. I'm simply saying that it is something you see that I don't. I don't know why that is.
- Sal, I only hear two voices in this room – yours and mine. I don't hear a woman's voice at all. What do you hear her say?
- Jamey, I know about the Democrats and the Republicans. I've never heard of the Illuminated Ones. I'm not arguing with you here. I'm just saying that I've never heard of them, so I'm not the person to talk about them.

Remember, the point here is not to convince the patient that their delusions are not real, or even that they are wrong. Your goal is to act respectfully, and not minimize or dismiss their viewpoint outright, something they regularly encounter.

Furthermore, differentiation keeps the lines of communication open. Think of two people from different cultures, or even two beings from different planets, trying to explain what it is like to live in their respective worlds. By maintaining a way that you can continue to talk, despite your differences, the patient is more likely to be open to you in other areas. If mentally ill people find themselves shut down or discounted when they try to talk about their perceptions or beliefs, it is very unlikely that they will be open to hospital staff about any other area of concern.

In some circumstances, you can act in concert with their belief without endorsing it. For example, you might say, "I can't see the laser beams, but I know lasers don't pass through solid objects. Maybe you will feel safer sitting in that room over there."[10]

Rule #7: Differentiate

You give the person the "right" to their own perceptions and beliefs. You inform them that you do not perceive what they do, but you are not arguing that *they* do not see it. In some cases, you can take their delusions into account without agreeing with them.

Steam Valve: When the Pressure Is Too Great

Some people, either with symptoms of psychosis or mania (Chapter 19), are so full of things to say, think, or feel that they seem like they are going to explode from the pressure. Words cascade out of them in floods of thought, in flights of ideas. Sometimes they make sense, but they totally dominate the "air time" in the room, and do not allow you to speak or to change the subject to something that must be attended to. At other times, they do not make sense at all. Their words may sound like poetry – "clang associations" – as they link words by sound, not by inherent meaning. They may jump from idea to idea in what are called "loose associations" or "tangential thinking."

Sometimes you simply have to say, with utmost kindness, "You have talked enough for awhile. It's time to be quiet. Hush." For some people, this works quite well for both sides. It is honest, it is direct, and it sets a limit.

At other times, one needs to let a little pressure off, like opening a valve in a steam pipe. Then you create space to say a bit of what you have to say. First, put out a hand, palm down, fingers curved at waist level – use this to interrupt. If they don't perceive it, put up both hands, using a little drama in your facial expression to get their attention and interrupt them. You let out a little pressure, so to speak, ask or say something, get a bit of information in return, and let them continue their cascade of ideas. You let out a little more pressure, and then once again, gently interrupt. Each time you speak, you show that you were listening – tracking what they say – sum it up a little, and then ask your question or make your statement.

As you see, *steam valving* is for the purpose of letting the person tell enough of what is pressuring him internally so that he does not fight you for the conversational floor. If you simply insist he stop talking about his delusions and then demand to know whether he's called his doctor and what they talked about, he may simply go silent or become more irrational as he perceives your frustration as frightening.

Example: Steam valving

Patient: "I was looking outside my window at the birdfeeder, and it was covered with goldfinches. The lemony yellow just burned my eyes so badly I closed the curtains. My eyes were burned by the fiery birds."

Staff person *(interrupting firmly)*: "Charles, I want to hear more about those birds. I haven't seen any goldfinches this year. But before you tell me more, I have a question. Did you call your doctor for an appointment?"

Patient: "Yes, I did, behind the closed drapes, where the birds couldn't burn my eyes out. I called and talked to a very nice nurse. They have a sound that is piercing to the brain, and a single glance can burn your eyes to a crisp. The birds, not the nurses."

Staff person: "I can see you are worried about your eyes. That's why you have the sunglasses, huh? I want you to tell me how the sunglasses are working, but first, what day is your appointment?"

Patient: "It's on a Thursday, but I don't know when, or what time. I'm burning among the birds, you see, with their lemony scalding flame."

Rule #8: Steam valve

This is useful for people whose speech is a cascade of words and ideas, often tangential or delusional. You listen and then tactfully but firmly interrupt. Sum up what the person says, tell them you want to hear more, but first you have a question to ask. On other occasions, you have an instruction to give, or something to tell the patient, and after they listen or comply, you let them return to their cascade of words. Listen a bit, then interrupt again. Remember, you must show in your response/interruption that you have been listening to what they say.

Structure and Predictability

Some people experiencing psychosis live in a world that seems about to fall into complete chaos. For others, it is frightening and unpredictable. One of the kindest things you can do is to help establish a sense of order. This can include trying to ensure that your office does not suddenly change in any drastic way, and that routines are done at the same hour on the same day. I am not suggesting that you make a clockwork environment in which every minute and every activity is timed. Nonetheless, when you work with people with psychosis, the world should become a familiar place, with few surprises. Whenever possible, prepare your patient well in advance when something new is going to happen, such as a new doctor, new clothes, or a new routine. Surprises are, for many people with psychosis, shocking experiences. When such advance notice cannot be given, you should use a low-key approach to introducing novelty, an approach that minimizes the "shock of the new" for your patient.

In either event, make your voice matter-of-fact. If you are too tentative and solicitous, they may think that something awful is going to happen and that is why you are talking in such careful tones. At the same time, do not affect a cheerful, "aren't-we-having-fun" tone of voice. Remember, the patient is anxious, even frightened. When you portray in your voice that it is "no big thing," you are, in effect, trivializing their very real concerns. Patronizing or belittling a patient will compromise their opportunity to make progress with their illness and may upset them enough that they react with more volatility when the fearful change occurs.

Rule #9: Structure and predictability

The more predictable and organized the environment around the person with psychosis, the safer they will feel.

Physical Space, Physical Contact, and the Use of the Eyes with Patients Experiencing Psychotic Symptoms

Be acutely aware when you are inadvertently "pressuring" the psychotic person by standing or sitting too close to them. Consider this *your* responsibility – do not expect the person to tell you of their discomfort. Indeed, the first sign that you are too close may be an assault. Sometimes, you can teach them either to speak up for themselves or to simply move away. But you should not add to their difficulties by looming over them or standing in such a way that they feel they cannot escape.

Other individuals who experience psychotic symptoms are not aware of personal space, and they may stand or sit too close to you. Firmly, without any harshness in your tone, tell them to move back: "Monty, I really want to hear what you are saying, but you are standing too close to me. I'd like you to take three steps back and then we can continue." Similarly, if a patient moves behind you, turn, make direct eye contact, and firmly tell them not to move behind you, that if they wish to talk with you, they should approach from the front.

Limit Setting is Assessment

Limit setting is a marvelous means of assessment. Consider the different responses a patient might make to your statement that they should not come up behind you:

- A blank, bewildered stare. They don't understand what you are talking about.
- Apologies. They are worried that you are mad at them because they did "something wrong."
- A sneer. "What's the matter? Are you paranoid or something? I just wanted to see the picture."
- A confrontation. "I can do what I want. You can't tell me how to live my life!"

For many individuals with psychosis, direct, sustained eye contact is the equivalent of physical contact or an intrusion into their personal space (Chapter 39). Mentally ill patients can misinterpret direct eye contact as aggressive, threatening, or seductive. Be aware of how your patients wish to be treated "visually." If they are uncomfortable with being looked at directly, occasionally "touch base" by making brief eye contact, then ease your eyes away, and then back again. <u>If, however, a patient is becoming aggressive, whether psychotic or not, direct eye contact is absolutely imperative</u>.

Physical contact presents the same dilemma as eye contact. For some, physical contact is obnoxious, confusing, over-exciting, or invasive – the possibilities are endless. Any physical contact is best kept to an absolute minimum. Of course, there is contact that is required by medical necessity, or in the event of assaultive behavior, physical restraint procedures. <u>Any time you are moved to make contact, beyond that, such as a comforting hand to the shoulder, you must be clear what clinical purpose, beyond your desire to be compassionate, for example, "demands" it.</u> Even when it clearly ***could be*** the right thing to do (for example, putting an arm around the shoulder of a distraught teenager who just got word that her dog died while she was hospitalized), that is still predicated upon whether your patient agrees. Some people, however, are too inarticulate, anxious, shy, or confused to express what they feel. Pay attention to the subtle information they often give you, sometimes in spite of themselves. You will often be quite able to tell if your patient welcomes or rejects a hand on the shoulder: by muscular tension, stiffening, pulling away, or other very clear physical signs. Other people, however, are so lost inside themselves that these reactions are hidden. Don't assume, then, that a lack of reaction means acceptance.

Rule #10: Body spacing, body contact, and eye contact

- Be aware of physical spacing: do not stand too close. If your patient stands too close to you, tactfully, but firmly tell him or her to move back. Similarly, tell people firmly not to walk up close behind you.
- Limit eye contact: most people with psychosis are made anxious by too direct eye contact, experiencing it as either a threat or a challenge.
- <u>Any physical contact, beyond medical necessity and protection from violence, is contingent on three things: hospital policy, clinical necessity, and patient wishes</u>. There are few occasions – outside children's programs – where you will be making much body contact with your patients, beyond medical interventions and physical restrain in the case of an assault or other imminent danger. Be absolutely sure that body contact – essentially a firm hand momentarily on the shoulder – is welcome AND that there is an absolutely clear clinical *necessity* for this contact.

CHAPTER 19

Welcome to the Rollercoaster:
Tactics for Dealing with
Symptoms of Mania

Mania is a state of high energy. Individuals who are manic usually require little sleep and are often excited, grandiose, agitated, or irritable. They may have flights of ideas, which can be either creative or completely irrational – or both at the same time. Their speech is often pressured: not only is it rapid, but also there is a sense that there is always more to say than they can get out, like water forcing its way through a too-narrow aperture. They are usually extremely confident, and this confidence is often accompanied by a sense of invulnerability. Not infrequently, these patients can also be selfish or narcissistic. They feel wonderful, and their own needs and desires are the only thing that matters. Their judgment can be extremely poor, and they engage in behaviors that can put them or others at risk.

The manic state is most commonly associated with bipolar disorder (manic-depressive disorder), in which periods of mania are interspersed with periods of depression. Some drugs can also cause manic episodes (particularly stimulant drugs such as methamphetamine or cocaine), and mania can be a side effect of psychiatric medications. People with traumatic brain injuries may exhibit periods of agitation that look very much like mania, but these episodes are often more extreme and disorganized than the classic manic state. On the other hand, manic people can get so agitated (manic excitement) that they shift into a delirium state. Whatever the cause, *delirious* individuals are de-escalated using the strategies for chaotic rage (Chapter 57).

Imagine a beautiful spring day: the sky is blue, birds are singing, and a gentle breeze is blowing. You wake up and leap out of bed, happy to be alive. You have so much energy that it is difficult to contain. When you think about the work you have to do today, it seems so easy: you will be finished in no time at all! You just know you will make some new friends today, maybe hook up with an attractive person and everything will click and you'll be in love or at least lust – so you are going to go to the park, the club, the bar, wherever, and enjoy life. <u>Imagine that feeling day-after-day, multiplied by ten- or twenty-fold</u>. Can you see how easy it would be to begin to make unwise choices, how your confidence could lead you to, for example, hijack that freight train because ever since you were a child, you wanted to be an engineer?[11]

When you feel this good, it seems like a good idea to feel *even better*. Thus, manic individuals very often turn to drugs and alcohol in order to "keep the good times rolling." Conversely, manic patients may also try to calm themselves with depressant drugs, such as barbiturates, heroin, and alcohol. Alcohol can have a "paradoxical effect" on some manic individuals, however, further exciting rather than sedating them.

Manic people often talk in rapid cascades of words, a waterfall of ideas leaping from one area to another. Sometimes you can follow their thoughts, although they are speaking very rapidly, but at other times, they leap and zigzag, making connections that have little or no meaning to you.

Manic energy often turns sexual, and the person may get involved with people who may be inappropriate or even dangerous for them.

They may spend money to buy anything and everything, running up their credit cards to the max.

Some patients with mania become very irritable, with a hair-trigger temper. They may also become provocative, teasing and taunting other people. Think of the dynamic portrayed in the Warner Brother cartoons of the Roadrunner and the Coyote. This may seem to be all in good fun at first, but it goes too far – way too far. Others may simply try to pick a fight. Because these patients so easily become angry or even violent, it is very important that you familiarize yourself with the latter sections in this book concerning de-escalation of anger and rage.

Finally, in extreme manic states, people can become psychotic, with all the symptoms of grandiosity, persecutory, paranoid, and religious delusions that any other psychotic individual might.

Brittle Grandiosity

Manic people can act or describe themselves as if they do not have a care in the world. They spin ideas, one after another, and expect both agreement and admiration. They seem utterly self-confident. Think of manic grandiosity, however, as a fragile structure, like a tower made of spun sugar. It glitters, it glows, and it's huge, but tap the wrong strut or beam, and the entire tower falls down in shards.

A healthy, self-confident individual can handle criticism or teasing easily; they are resilient. Unfair criticisms are met with a gracious laugh or a dignified response. The manic person, on the other hand, if teased for their somewhat irrational ideas, can misinterpret this as an attack, thinking they are being made fun of. Any criticisms or perceived teasing may be met with sudden aggression or rage. In other words, consider the manic flight of words to be a kind of hysteria. Even when these patients appear happy, it is as if they were on a giddy flight hanging onto a helium balloon. Miscalculated teasing or criticism is experienced as if you are poking at the balloon with a needle.

Humor can occasionally be a useful form of communication with such patients. But you need to be calm and centered (Section IV). Even if you say something that is funny, <u>your purpose must be to catch</u>

their attention and slow things down, not to have fun with them. Trying to *match* wits with them is like trying to catch a dragonfly in flight. Help them down to earth instead.

Watch Out! Mania Can Be Infectious

Being with these patients can be very exciting, particularly if they are at low or moderate levels of escalation. They can be brilliant conversationalists: witty, sexy, provocative, and entertaining. It can be like having your own comedian – fast on their feet, bawdy, and full of fun. We can easily catch their mood. It is easy to begin to feel grandiose and over-confident ourselves. But hitching a ride on this energy is just as dangerous in the hospital as it would be on the highway: once you've jumped in the back seat and are zigzagging down the road at 90 miles an hour, it's pretty hard to get back out of the vehicle.

Patients with mania assume that you are in absolute agreement with them when you "hitch a ride." They have a sense of union with you and think that what they want is what you want. They assume that their actions and behaviors, no matter how noncompliant, are acceptable. However, when you subsequently set any kind of limit on those behaviors, the manic patient may suddenly turn on you in betrayed anger.

It is absolutely paramount, from your initial contact, that you firmly establish a solid professional relationship with the manic patient, with clear-cut limits. This must continue among all staff and the patient throughout their stay in the hospital. Manic individuals can be very manipulative while appearing to be friendly and engaging. Remember, the manic patient may be very provocative, trying to set you up for an overreaction or making you look like a fool. They often sexualize interactions: you must be very cautious that they do not perceive sexual interest on your part based on your letting pass some innuendo or mild flirtatious comment.

The expression "He's a drag" refers to someone who slows the party down. That is not a bad idea with these patients.

- Stay centered.
- Do not get swept away or swept up in their energy.
- Focus on slowing things down. Speak slower, and take things step-by-step.

The Medication Struggle: It's NOT Like Diabetes

As stated earlier, mania is a unique state in that one feels wonderful, healthy, confident, and effective, but is actually not doing well at all. If the mania is due to drug abuse, of course people must stop using if they are to heal. If the mania is due to a medication side effect, then they must see a doctor.

When the problem is caused by bipolar disorder, medication can usually control the symptoms. However, some bipolar folks believe, in some ways correctly, that they will feel worse when they take the medications. Yes, perhaps they will be calm and more organized, sleep more hours, and not get in as much trouble. They may also avoid crushing periods of depression. However, life will lose a wonderful glow, and the hours of each day will be more like lead than gold. Unlike almost any other condition, profoundly "ill" patients often feel best when they are most ill. People with bipolar illness will resist taking medication unless their lives on medication are rich and interesting, so much so that they are willing to spurn the dangerous wonders that the manic state seems to offer.

When encouraging a bipolar person to take medications, many professionals and family members say, "It's a condition like diabetes. You need to take it every day to maintain yourself. It's not like medicine for a sore throat that you take until you are cured, and then never have to take again." Although this is true, there is a very profound difference between diabetes and bipolar disorder. If you do not take your medicine for diabetes, you very quickly become seriously ill, and you feel awful too. If people with bipolar disorder discontinue medication, they often feel much better than when they were taking it. Therefore, it is far better to focus your discussion on the important aspects of these patients' lives *while* they are on medication. In short, ordinary medicated life should be tangibly better *to them* than the un-medicated carnival of the manic state. If not, it is very unlikely that your patient will be med-compliant.

Review: Interacting with the manic individual

You will recognize the manic person because they will display super high energy. They will often talk very fast, and their ideas will "zigzag" from one to another. They often act like comedians, with a rapid-fire delivery. Their behavior may also be either sexualized or hair-trigger aggressive. In either case, they will also be provocative.

- Remain calm and centered.
- Be conscious of the patient's brittle grandiosity, a fragile state of mind, in spite of his or her claims to the contrary. Grandiose does not mean strong!
- Do not bluntly criticize.
- Do not tease or joke around. If you use any humor, it is for the purpose of slowing them down, not having fun.
- Try to enforce compliance with their medications. At the same time, the metaphor linking diabetes and other chronic illnesses with bipolar disorder is often useless. Develop individualized strategies that resonate with the patient, highlighting the wonders of the medicated, well-ordered, and productive life. If the patient does not desire this life, they will usually be noncompliant with medication regimens.

CHAPTER 20

Communication and De-escalation
with Elderly Patients

Effectively working with elderly patients, particularly if they are mentally disabled, is one of the most challenging situations you might face. Nonetheless, you must remember that older adults are not a monolithic category. They are people – like all of us – simply older. Every character type, every mode of aggression, every mental syndrome, and every de-escalation strategy applies to elderly people as well as to those of other age groups. Despite their age, elderly people do assault others, particularly caregivers. Their rage can emerge from confusion, medical conditions, pain, adverse drug mental illness, pure meanness or hate, or any number of stressors. The following, which have both human and tactical value, should be considered:

- Be aware that elderly people may be resistant to help. This may be due to disorganization, confusion brought on by dementia, a combination of severe depression and fear, or pride ("At least I still have the strength to refuse someone.").
- Speak respectfully, befitting the age and seniority of the person. Too many people speak to the elderly in a patronizing, demeaning tone.
- Use their honorific and last name unless specifically invited to use their first name. If you wish to achieve a more informal relationship, ask, "Would you prefer to be called Mrs. X or by your first name?" Let them *offer* the first name.
- When it is not an immediately emergent situation, take a little bit more time. Attempt to "nibble around the edges," talking about life, about family. Be aware, however, that many elderly people have lost everyone in their lives.
- Be prepared to get enormously frustrated at their leaden stubbornness, that "the person simply won't do what is good for them." What appears as inertia, however, may be a profound expression of fear. Remember that the most proximate change that many elderly people are concerned with is death; in states of confusion or fear, any situation provoking anxiety evokes the fear of death. You may think they are defiant – but they may be scared out of their wits.
- Do not talk around or about the person to others as if they are not there.
- Do not barrage them with choices, decisions, or too much information.
- Paranoia (Chapter 10), whatever the cause, is one of the frequent triggers of rage in elderly people – particularly those with dementia or adverse drug reactions. As the person becomes suspicious, you can often change the subject so that the object of their suspicion recedes from their awareness.
- The rage and violence that emerges with elderly people is frequently chaotic. Please refer to Chapter 14 regarding communication with disorganized people and Chapter 57 on de-escalation of people in chaotic states.

A responsibility to learn restraint procedures appropriate to elderly people

The reader may be an employee from a psychiatric hospital or care facility in which physical restraint is used to ensure safety for the violent patient, other patients, and staff. Because of the particular vulnerabilities of elderly people, your physical restraint instructors should consult with medical specialists, particularly paramedics and emergency medical technicians, regarding what type of physical guidance and restraint offers the least risk of injury to elderly patients. This should be integrated into your training scenarios.

SECTION IV

Centering: Standing with
Strength and Grace
in Crisis Situations

CHAPTER 21

Introduction to Centering

The first three sections of this book focus on behaviors of patients that, at minimum, make them difficult to communicate with, and in more severe situations, are manifestations of impaired cognitive functioning and/or emotional regulation. These chapters approach the subjects with a degree of clinical distance: the behavior is described, and tactics are suggested to best communicate with such people.

However, de-escalation is not merely a matter of assessment and technical skill. Who *you* are and how you behave is absolutely crucial to establishing a peaceful interaction with your patients. Without a sense of centering and calm, it is impossible to assist other people in calming themselves. The strategies in this section revolve around maintaining self-control. For many of us, "control" implies something forceful and rigid. On the contrary, we should aim to develop the ability to adapt to circumstances in a powerful, fluid, and purposeful way. Not only will this enhance your ability to work with your patients on a day-to-day basis, but it will also make you most effective in crisis situations. Sometimes you quietly listen, and other times you quickly intervene. You are not defensive or on your guard. Rather, like a cat walking along a fence, you are at ease, yet ready for anything that comes. At the same time, you are equally prepared to escape or, in a worst-case scenario, fight back.

Example: Preparing for the worst while presenting the best of oneself

I was once asked to do an outreach to the apartment of a severely mentally ill man, suffering from schizophrenia. His mother had not been seen for several weeks, and due to his long history of violence, people were concerned about her well-being. Approximately six months before, he had half-bitten off the nose of a law enforcement officer during a violent struggle.

I knocked on the door, with two police officers hiding on either side of the entrance, their hands on their guns. The man opened the door with his teeth literally bared. His face with twisted in an amalgam of rage and fear, and he stared into my eyes with the anguished look of a trapped prisoner.

I stood several arms' lengths away, and I gave a slight bow, saying, "I am so sorry to bother you. I know you didn't expect to see me at your door. I have just a couple of questions, and as soon as you answer them, I will leave right away. The first question is, where is your mother?"

He jumped a little and after a long pause replied, "At my aunt's house."

"Thank you. My second question is, can I have her phone number?"

He backed up, hand out, and said, "You wait here. You wait here." A moment later, he returned with a piece of paper, with a phone number written on it. He reached out to hand it to me, his eyes wild. With no way of knowing if my moving would frighten him or if he was trying to reach out to grab me, I held up my hands and said, "That's OK. You hold it up for me and I'll write it down from here. You probably want to keep that number."

I wrote the number on my hand and said, "Thank you. That's all. Good-bye." He rocked back and forth in the entry way and then closed the door. The officers and I walked down the hall, checking behind us just to be sure, and then, outside the building, heaved a collective sigh of relief.

This incident exemplifies what I am trying to convey in this section. Here are the main components of my interaction with the man that almost surely averted an assault:

- I breathed smoothly and calmly. This kept me calm, and furthermore, there was nothing in my body language that suggested to the man that I wanted to fight him.
- I was acutely aware of physical spacing. I maintained spacing that did not pressure him, and also was as safe for myself as I could establish under the circumstances.
- I was ready for the worst while presenting the best of myself. I had an empathic sense of the man's fear, and although somewhat frightened of him myself (this fear is common sense – simply an awareness that one is in a potentially dangerous situation), I treated him with respect and decency.

If any of the readers are wondering, I did call the aunt's house, and the man's mother was safe.

CHAPTER 22

"I've Got All the Time I Need":
Hurrying Slowly

When your patients are in crisis, they believe that there is no time and no hope to solve the problem. If you agree, you, too, are in crisis. Instead, you must have an attitude that, no matter what, you have all the time you need to find an answer to the problem. Whether the other person agrees or not is not the question. The answer must start within you.

We cannot make a mentally ill or drug-abusing person "better." It is as if we are standing by the bank of a river at flood, and there is a person in the water, drowning. If we dive in to save them, they will try to climb on top of us to reach just a little more air, causing us both to drown. Instead, we must remain on the bank, skillfully throwing a rope. We point to it and encourage the drowning person to take hold. Were we to throw too quickly, we'd miss them or end up with a tangle of cord, elaborate but useless. Instead, "hurrying slowly," we cast it with studied grace. We can pull them up, however, only if they grab the rope. If they refuse, there is nothing we can do. Our best hope that they will take hold is if we are calm and *passionately dispassionate*. When we convey a sense of warm, confident gravity, we pass to the other person the sense that we *both* have all the time we need.

CHAPTER 23

It's Not Personal Unless
You Make It So

The brain is an organ of survival. It is organized to respond to threat. We are aware of danger through pattern recognition, a rapid response of the more primitive areas of the brain. A large object moving rapidly towards us, a sudden pain, or a violent grab initiates a cascade of actions – fight/flight/freeze/faint – that are expressed to keep us alive in the worst of circumstances. At lower levels of danger, particularly those presented by another human being, we are provoked into posturing – dominance/submission displays – which are attempts to maintain or enhance our position in a social structure.

The curse of being human, however, is that these survival responses are precipitated by noxious stimuli that elicit physiological responses, particularly that which shocks or surprises us. When our brain perceives these responses, it responds as if we are in life-threatening danger, even when that is not the case.

In the heat of an argument, people sometimes say things in desperation that they later regret. Other times, they deliberately hone in on a person's weak spot. They say things that feel like a dagger to the gut. We feel beaten or raped by the words that are being said, and we cannot make our attacker stop.

Sometimes your patients will challenge you by trying to offend you or by making you explain yourself. Provocative challenges are for the purpose of getting leverage on you. By weakening you, the other person feels more personal power. However, verbal abuse is not really dangerous to you, except the risk that you will lose control of your own actions, thus fueling further conflict between you.

Rule 1: I don't have to agree that we are in an argument

A desire to win an argument is associated with primitive mental processes linked to dominance hierarchies. Rather than striving for the truth or for an equitable exchange, we end up striving to overwhelm the other. Unless you are in a struggle for your life, <u>you do not have to win</u>. Your goal should be to establish peace between the two of you.

Rule 2: I don't have to give back what I get

We believe ourselves justified when we counterattack because they "hurt us first." However, a defensive reaction or move toward revenge is another manifestation of an attempt to assert dominance over the other. Striking back is an attempt to wound. When patients hurt your feelings because of what they say or do, remember that <u>it is an act of valor not to respond in kind</u>.

Rule 3: It's not personal

Realize that although their attacks on you might seem personal, that is only so when you make it so. If the attack is untrue, what is there to be upset about? And if what they say is valid, then you are reacting in anger when someone tells you the truth: you knew it already, so what is there to be upset about?

Bracketing: Naming Your Hot Buttons

The trouble with the three rules above is that they work fine until we get our buttons pushed. When our buttons are pushed, we react as if we are threatened with bodily harm: this reaction, in most cases, ill serves the reestablishment of peace.

Bracketing is a method of mastering ourselves through mastering our reactions to our buttons. Bracketing means facing our vulnerabilities head on and making a firm resolve that no one will use them against us. This is not easy to do. It takes courage to look closely at yourself and say, "These are my areas of greatest vulnerability." In a spiritual sense, you must strip yourself utterly naked and face yourself as you truly are. Doing so, however, will give you the greater strength that self-knowledge always brings. NOT doing so will make you more vulnerable to the attacks of your patients.

You might think that talking about your vulnerabilities with a friend could help you to stay truthful and strong. However, talking about such difficult issues with another person often results in them trying to reassure or comfort you, reframing the "bad" as "not so bad," or giving you an excuse to explain why you are the way you are. To really identify your vulnerabilities, you must face the worst without the refuge of a comforting friend or witness.

It is important, therefore, to look deeply within yourself and identify what your buttons are. Buttons come in five primary "colors":

- I can't stand it when someone attacks or demeans <   >, because that's something I love and treasure.
- I feel outraged when someone demeans <   > because it is something I believe to be unquestionably right and good.
- People get me defensive when they say or point out <   >, because, to tell the truth, I hate it in myself.
- When people say or do <   >, I lose it because it's as if they are taking control of me, or disrespecting me.
- They better not say <   >. That's the one word I won't take from anyone.

Statement	Why does this get to me?
EXAMPLE: When people say or do < >, I lose it because	

Taking Inventory

Not surprisingly, we are most likely to lose our temper (our flexibility and strength) when we are blindsided. Sudden emotional shock elicits the same responses in the nervous system as a physical attack. For example, if someone you trust suddenly insults your race, religion, or gender, you will likely respond using the part of your brain that expresses raw emotion. This part of the brain is not concerned about the truth, about negotiation, or about a past history of friendship. Instead, it views the world as one at war, with the other person trying to destroy one's position of strength.

To avoid this, take inventory. <u>Every morning, upon waking, and even a few more times during the day, run through those flaws you just enumerated above</u>. The idea is the same as checking the gas, mirrors, and lights on your car before leaving your driveway. When (not "if") a patient – or coworker – tries to push one of your buttons, you are not surprised or caught off guard. You expect it without being anxious about it. If you take inventory, you center yourself for another day, ready for the worst without it tearing you down.

People often fool themselves about being centered. It is radically different from merely being "relaxed" or "open." Being centered is a dynamic, active state: like a cat on a fence, not a cow standing in a field. This does not mean that you are at hair-trigger readiness, something closer to paranoia than mindful grace. Rather, you develop a sense of spaciousness, in tune with your surroundings and your emotions. Although not *particularly* expecting an attack, you are not surprised either, because you are used to reminding yourself where you can be hurt. Because you are no longer as vulnerable, you will find it easier to take control of a critical incident when you are needed. You will also find that you can disengage and walk away from a situation when that's the right thing to do. When you really know your buttons, you will not be blindsided. Your insecurities and weaknesses are still present, but you have control over them.

In essence, you should resolve each day that no one will "drag you down." The only thing that you will take personally is your own dignity.

CHAPTER 24

Circular Breathing:
Be the Eye in the Center
of the Hurricane

Violence, disputes, and arguments can sweep through one's daily routine with the suddenness and force of a hurricane. Your previously calm day can become chaotic, and worse, you may feel that chaos will overwhelm you too. But, when you can step coolly into the worst of situations, you embody the eye of the hurricane, with all the chaos coalescing and revolving around you. The root of this skill lies in breath control. When you breathe slowly, with focused attention, you regain control of your physical self. When you control your body, you control your life. Then you are in a position to take control of the crisis – and the person causing it.

Two Variations

Circular breathing is derived from East Asian martial traditions and was used to keep warriors calm on the battlefield. There are two variations of circular breathing. Try both, alternating between them, until you know which one works best for you. Then, exclusively practice the one you prefer. At the initial stages, practice circular breathing sitting in a comfortable position, in a peaceful environment. Once you master this breathing method, it can be used in any environment, with any body posture. *If you train regularly, it will kick in automatically, rather than being something you must think about.* In essence, your breath itself becomes your center: not your body posture, not the situation in which you find yourself, or the quality of the relationship you may have with the patient.

Breathing for crisis, not bliss

Lest there be any confusion: This is NOT a "time-out" where you take a few deep breaths and then return to the subject, refreshed. There's no time for that in a crisis. On the contrary, you can be moving very fast while breathing very slowly. You are training your body and mind to go into this breathing as a response to danger and stress, a trained response that should be instantaneous.

As someone who has practiced the following technique for over thirty years, I can assert that it has become automatic. Unlike in my younger days when the adrenalin would hit and I'd start breathing fast and high in the chest, now my breathing usually slows down in emergency situations. You are practicing to develop a "pseudo-instinct" – a trained response so bone-deep that you do not even have to think about it, anymore than you have to tell yourself to yank your hand from a hot stove.

Circular Breathing Method #1

- Sit comfortably, feet on the floor, hands in your lap.
- Sit relaxed, but upright. Do not slump or twist your posture.
- Keep your eyes open. (As you practice, so you will do.) If you practice with your eyes closed, your newly trained nervous system will send an impulse to close your eyes in emergency situations. If you want to use a breathing method for closed-eye guided imagery or relaxation – to get *away* from your problems, so to speak – use another method altogether.
- Breathe in through the nose.
- Imagine the air traveling in a line down the front of your body to a point 2 inches below the navel.
- Momentarily pause, letting the breath remain in a dynamic equilibrium.
- Without straining or holding the breath, exhale through your nose.
- As you exhale, imagine the air looping around your lower body, between your legs and up through the base of your spine.
- As you continue to exhale, imagine the air going up your spine and around your head and then out of your nose.

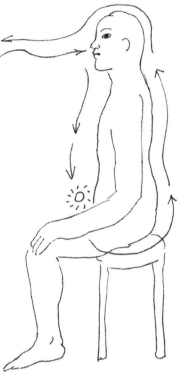

Circular Breathing Method #2

- Sit comfortably, feet on the floor, hands in your lap.
- Sit relaxed, but upright. Do not slump or twist your posture.
- Keep your eyes open. (As you practice, so you will do.) If you practice with your eyes closed, your newly trained nervous system will send an impulse to close your eyes in emergency situations. If you want to use a breathing method for closed-eye guided imagery or relaxation – to get *away* from your problems, so to speak – use another method altogether.
- Breathe in through the nose.
- Imagine the air around the head, looping down the back, falling down each vertebrae, continuing down past the base of the spine to the perineum, and looping again, this time up the front of the body to a point 2 inches below the navel.
- Momentarily pause, letting the breath remain in a dynamic equilibrium.
- Without straining or holding the breath, exhale through your nose.
- As you exhale, imagine the air ascending up the centerline of your body and out your nose.

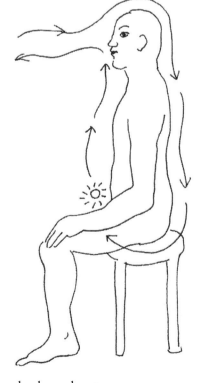

How to Practice Circular Breathing

Some people find it helpful to imagine that their breath has light or color. Others take a finger or object to trace a line down and around the centerline of the body to help focus their attention. Choose which of the variations works better for you.

When you first practice, do so while seated and balanced. Once you develop some skill, try circular breathing while standing, leaning, or even driving. You will soon be able to use this breathing in any posture and under any circumstance. Most people find that after a short time they do not need to visualize the circulation of the breath. You literally will feel it, a ring of energy running through your body. You begin to feel balanced and ready for anything.

Once you are comfortable with your chosen pattern of breathing, experiment with it in slightly stressful circumstances, like being caught in traffic or stuck in the supermarket checkout line, with the person in front of you painstakingly counting out change and coupons. Try it also when afflicted with anxiety – stage fright, a meeting with your supervisor, or a patient who always seems to put you off balance. When you can better manage yourself in these slightly aggravating or anxiety-provoking situations, you are ready to use it in a crisis situation. If you have practiced enough, you will naturally shift into this mode of breathing when you find yourself in a crisis. There will no longer be a need to tell yourself to "do" circular breathing. It will become reflexive, automatic, replacing old patterns of breathing that actually increased anxiety or anger within you.

Remember, this is a skill to use during emergencies, not for relaxation or meditative purposes. Instead, you are trying to develop an "omni-directional potential energy." You are ready to fight, to dodge, to leave, to think gracefully and intelligently, whatever is required for the situation at hand.

When Should You Use Circular Breathing?

The way you physically organize affects your thinking. For example, if you assumed the posture and breathing of a depressed person (slumped body, shallow breathing, sighing), and maintained it awhile, you'd actually start to feel depressed. Similarly, if you clenched your fists and started glaring around you with a lot of tension in your body, you'd start to feel angry. (You have probably observed a number of individuals working themselves up from anger through rage into an attack in just this way.) Circular breathing is used to create a professional mind-set, one adaptable and ready for anything, equally prepared for an easy conversation or for a fight, yet fixed on neither.

This method of breathing is very helpful when you are anticipating a crisis situation, perhaps when you are expecting a troublesome individual to visit the hospital or preparing to deliver some bad news. This breathing activates the entire nervous system in a way that enhances both creativity and the ability to survive.

Even in the middle of a confrontation, particularly a verbal one, there are many times when this breathing will have a very powerful effect. Not only do we get more stressed or upset in the presence of an upset person, but we also become more peaceful in the presence of a calm one. People tend to template their mood to the most powerful individual close by. Think of a staff person you know who, when they walk onto a scene, often calms it down before they've said a word. You've probably seen the opposite as well. Using this breathing method is a vital tool in making you the former type, a man or woman of quiet power.

You should use this method of breathing after the crisis is resolved as well. A crisis does not usually occur at the end of the day, and you will need to regroup in order to go on with your job. Circular breathing will bring you back to a calm and relaxed state, prepared to handle the next crisis, should one occur.

Circular breathing will also prevent you from carrying the crisis back home with you at the end of the day. Before entering your home, sit quietly in your car or yard and practice circular breathing for a moment or two. The only thing that should come home is you, not the crises you weathered.

Breathing for Healing from Trauma or Warding off Traumatic Reactions

Circular breathing, along with a particular method of imagery work, is an effective method of warding off the effects of potentially traumatic events.

Post-traumatic stress is not defined by how horrible the event sounds in description, by the victim's response to the event. PTSD is not exactly a problem of memory – it is a problem because the event has not fully *become* a memory – the event is still primarily experienced as if it were happening right now. When an event is fully a memory, it is experienced as something in the past, over and done with. Or think of it as a scar: it may not be pretty, and it certainly is a signpost that something significant happened, but it no longer hurts. A trauma, on the other hand, is an open wound. It is an *experience.* It is not in the past, and it may be affecting every moment of the person's life; or it may emerge suddenly, when evoked by something that elicits a sense that the event is happening again.

In PTSD, the person's nervous system is set to react as if there is an emergency whenever the trauma is recalled. This can be anything from an explicit memory to a small reminder: for example, although he does not consciously know why, a soldier gets anxious every time someone coughs, because one of his squad coughed right before a bomb went off. Because trauma affects the brain at the deepest levels associated with survival, logical interventions (anything from reassurance to cognitive therapy) offer only equivocal success in helping people emerge from trauma. Image-associated breathing techniques, which affect the brain as a whole, can assist people in realizing that the event is over, no longer a part of present experience.

How to Do Imagery-associated Breath Work
- Let us imagine that something very upsetting has happened to you. Perhaps you even recall an old trauma that still plagues your mind.
- Whenever you think about it (or it forcibly intrudes into your consciousness), your body tenses or twists in various ways. Your breathing pattern often changes.

- If this is your situation, go someplace where you will not be disturbed for a while. Make the mental image of that trauma as vivid as you can tolerate. This takes some courage, because most of us simultaneously avoid-as-we-remember. Rather, if only for a moment or two, meet it head on and re-experience it. If you physically organize *as if* something is happening, the brain believes that it truly is. Notice, in fine detail, how you physically and emotionally react. As difficult as this may be, it is important to establish for yourself a baseline response to the trauma. We must clearly experience what it "does" to us.

- Now take a couple of deep sighs. Sighing breaks up patterns of muscular tension and respiration. This is like rebooting your computer when the program is corrupt.

- Mentally say to the ugly experience, "Hush. You move right over there to my right (or left). I'll get to you in a minute." For some people, it is even helpful to make a physical gesture, "guiding" or "pushing" the experience off to the side. We cannot *force* ourselves to stop thinking about an experience if it has psychological power. Instead, we move it aside, as if we are guiding a wounded person to a waiting room while we organize ourselves to properly deal with it.

- Now initiate your preferred method of circular breathing.

- As the memory creeps back in (and it will), just breathe and center yourself, again placing the memory off to the side. Once again say, "Hush, I'll get to you in a minute." You can't fight it, so don't try. Just ease it aside until you are ready.

- When your breathing is smooth and your body is centered, you will be relaxed like an athlete, ready to move but with no wasted effort.

- Now, deliberately bring that ugly memory or trauma into your thoughts and imagination. As you find yourself reacting, continue circular breathing, trying to bring yourself back to physical balance as you focus on the traumatic memory.

- Bit by bit, in either one session or a few, you will notice that you are increasingly able to hold the image with a relaxed body and a balanced posture. You are now able to re-experience the memory without the same painful, tense, or distorted response you used in the past. You are, metaphorically speaking, turning the open wound into scar tissue.

Think of how you hold babies so that they are safe: you do not drop or squeeze them so tightly that they are frightened or uncomfortable. To be strong in the face of trauma is very similar in that you internally hold the memory with all the gentle strength with which you hold babies so that they are safe, whether asleep or struggling to see over your shoulder. You are not wiping the slate of memory clean. Rather, you are placing it in a proper context: it is something that happened to you, but it does not define you.

Cautions:

- Until you master the breathing as a pure act, you cannot use it as a tool to deal with trauma. <u>Furthermore, until you can do this for yourself, you *cannot* teach it to patients</u>. This truly is a skill that you can only lead the way by experience.

- Do not do trauma work of this kind with patients unless you have both training and experience in working with trauma survivors.

- If you are working with someone who is seriously traumatized, it will be better to have the person do the breath work in your presence.
- Ensure that the patient has mastered circular breathing and can use it to manage day-to-day stressors before trying to use it for trauma work. Do not ask your patient to do something beyond his or her capabilities.
- If "facing" the trauma is overwhelming, the patient can focus on one sense at a time: what they heard, smelled, saw, or felt.
- Have the patient focus on the trauma very briefly, and then breathe through the momentary flash of emotion and re-experiencing of the trauma. Do this several times, as if dipping one's toe in very cold water, gradually getting acclimated to it, rather than plunging in headfirst.

A particular value of circular breathing imagery work – doing for yourself

If, on a daily basis, you can "inoculate" yourself against stressful, even potentially traumatic experiences, life will continue to be enjoyable or will become enjoyable once again, even as you continue to work in a highly stressful environment. You will begin to develop what author David Grossman calls a "bulletproof mind." The goal is not to restore some kind of mythic "innocence" that you had "pre-trauma." The goal is to relegate the experience to its proper place: something ugly that happened sometime in the past but in no way controls the present.

CHAPTER 25

The Intoxication and Joy
of Righteous Anger

Most people consider anger to be a harmful emotion, one that upsets the angry person as well as the recipient. But this is not true for everyone. Some people, who are neither cruel nor hurtful, do not mind fighting in the least, particularly when they believe their cause is just. Such individuals go off-center in an interesting way – they get calm, even happy, when someone offends them. Perhaps they get a smile and mentally say, "If you want trouble, you came to the right place." As a boxer once told me, "When he [my opponent] gets hurt, he wants the round to be over. When I get hurt, I get happy."

Such people, when functioning in a professional capacity, have an especially difficult task – they must recognize that when they feel *good*, they are in danger of becoming part of the problem. Instead of imposing calm on a situation, they flame it up, and don't mind in the least. The person they are dealing with is a transgressor and the "happy warrior" feels completely righteous in responding in kind.

Circular breathing (Chapter 24), for those who are anxious, stressed, or frightened, provides a real sense of peace and relief. However, if confrontation feels good to you, such calming breathing seems like the last thing you would like to do. You think, "Center myself? Hell, no. I'm right where I want to be."

If this description fits, your task is to recognize the special joy that comes with righteous anger and act to center yourself to a calm state of mind, even though in the heat of the moment, it feels like a loss rather than a gain.

> **Example: Some people evoke conflict**
> There are times when you are responding to an angry patient, and you see several staff persons coming to back you up and at the sight of one of them, you think, "Oh, Lord, this is not going to go well!" They are exactly where they want to be; angry yet safe, especially because there are other staff around. They become indignant and self-righteous and escalate the situation the moment they hit the scene. Other staff, with no intention of provoking a confrontation, walk into the situation with a particular attitude that ticks everyone off, patients and other staff alike.

The righteously angry staff person may be known for this type of reaction. He or she is the one most likely to *not* recognize this, and *not* believe they need to do any breathing or calming. If this is you, recognize it! If this is a coworker, alert them to this flaw in their skills, if you have a close enough relationship to do so. If not, alert your supervisor, because this type of attitude puts other patients and staff at severe risk.

This is not about becoming some sort of Zen sage, never angered, never off-balance. Of course, you will be angry. In many situations you should be angry. It may even keep you alive. The problem is when anger justifies anything from treating aggravating or troublesome patients with contempt to actions that are overly harsh, clinically inappropriate, or even unethical on the extreme edge.

Protecting family from what we otherwise would bring home

Another type of righteous anger is that evoked when someone does something so clearly wrong that one feels annihilation of the perpetrator is the only justifiable response. Returning to the subject of the last chapter, this is a particularly important example of how such breathing can protect your family. At various times in my career, I have had the experience of feeling utterly contaminated by being in the presence of the perpetrators of child abuse or sexual assault. In the course of your responsibilities in the hospital where you work, you may have similar encounters. Speaking for myself, there have been times where I have felt a failure for treating the patient in a professional manner, a part of me feeling the right thing to do would be to grab them by the throat and start squeezing until they could never commit harm again.

Notwithstanding our horror or rage at what the person is alleged to have done, we must, of course, maintain our professionalism. Doing so, however, takes a toll. Therefore, beyond what I had to do on the job, I also made absolutely sure that I never brought such negative feelings home.

Instead, I would sit in my car in the driveway, using circular breathing to the breath around my body, maybe even going to a quiet place in the house or yard and working through the images in my brain so that when I walked into the presence of my wife and children, the only thing that ever entered my home was myself. No child molester or other evil-doer will ever walk into the house with me.

Beyond the protection of my family in this manner, this really helped me prevent burnout. Because I did not bring such feelings into my house, it remained a haven of love and peace, uncontaminated by the occasionally horrible things I encountered. Therefore, every morning I awoke restored, with strength to face the worst, because I kept it from infecting the fine things in my life.

CHAPTER 26

The Texture of Relationship and the Training of Intuition

The Spaces between Us

When a patient starts to become agitated or stressed, verbal exchanges are best kept simple. The patient will experience your elaboration of subtle therapeutic nuances, complicated case plans, or a financial program as confusing, aggravating, or threatening. The amount of physical space between you, the positioning of your hands and theirs, muscular tension, and the quality of your voice during those dangerous times – all those nonverbal expressions – become more important to the aggressive individual than what is actually being said.

There have been entire books written that attempt to codify the "language" of nonverbal communication. Although some of these works have excellent information, you will find little information relevant to the recognition of potentially dangerous people. Furthermore, there is a fair amount of nonsense published about "body language." Nonverbal behaviors are often idiosyncratic: not only do your patients have their own ways of physically expressing their emotions, but they also have their own ways of interpreting (or misinterpreting) yours. There is no checklist that will give you all the information you need to keep yourself and others safe.

It is crucial that we hone our ability to use intuition to pick up the warning signs that a dangerous situation is developing. Intuition is often experienced as mysterious. We seem to we know something without knowing exactly how we know it.

However, contrary to the belief that it is magic, mysticism, or luck, intuition can be trained. The best way to learn how to use and improve your intuitive ability is to study interpersonal space. Let us use the image of a bubble as a way of thinking about the shifting edges of one's personal space.[12] The space between us tends to expand and contract depending on the circumstances. For example, the more relaxed you are in the company of someone, the less personal space you require. When you are uncertain or suspicious of someone, you instinctively move to get more distance from them. Our mood can radically affect our sense of personal space: on a good day, you welcome people close to you, while on a bad mood day, you may need more space to tolerate others' proximity.

Space, however, is not just a matter of feet and inches. The space between human beings has a kind of "texture," something we apprehend by both physical responses and emotional reactions. If you enhance your ability to read and respond to the *quality* of that textured space, you will, by definition, begin to bring intuition under your conscious control.

Experiment 1: Practice Finding the Bubble

1. Ask a coworker or another trustworthy person who is willing to practice with you to stand in front of you, much farther away than he or she would ordinarily be while engaging in a normal conversation.

2. This person (the "sender") then begins to talk about a hobby, their family, or something that you are interested in.

3. As the sender talks, have him or her move toward you, slowly and easily. *There should not be any physical contact between you in this exercise.*

4. As the sender continues to talk and move toward you, you (the "receiver") are to become aware of the moment when the sender is too close for comfort – when he or she stepped into your bubble.

5. When that moment comes, hold up a hand and tell your practice partner to stop.

6. Now debrief this experience. Ask the sender or other observers to state whether they could tell by your body language that the sender was in fact in your bubble before you held up your hand. Have the sender describe how he or she knew this. This awareness is usually due to "tells" – physical behaviors that indicate discomfort or simply that the person is in your space. These behaviors can include stiffening, glazed eyes, tension, swaying back, or a fixed stare, to name of a few.

7. You then describe the physical sensation(s) that told you the sender was in your space. This sensation is your early warning sign that someone has trespassed your boundary. It is important not to confuse "physical sensation" with what we usually call "feelings" or "emotions," the *interpretation* of physical sensations and cognitions. Let us consider a "hollow feeling" in the belly. For one person, this means fear, and for another anticipation. A third may interpret this as excitement. Although such discussion may be interesting in its own right, we are only concerned here with the actual physical sensation that occurs within you when someone enters into your personal space.[13]

Experiment 2: Exploring the Texture of Relationship

Now try the same exercise, but have your partner try to con you or convince you to do something you don't want to do.

Observe whether you desire more or less space between you. Pay attention to your physical sensations in these circumstances. In what ways are they the same as your baseline experience (#1) and in what ways are they different?

Experiment 3: Pushing the Edges

Try it one more time with the sender yelling at you. This should not be an *overly* aggressive or frightening role-play exercise. Your practice partner, for example, could just pretend to be upset because you were late. (There should be no physical contact in this exercise: it is not a simulation of a violent encounter).

Study whether you desire for more or less space. Take some time to reflect on your physical sensations. In what ways are they the same as your baseline experience (#1) and in what ways are they different?

Experiment 4: Reading Your Partner's Bubble

Now reverse roles. You become the sender and your partner is the receiver.

Repeat the above exercises and watch the other person's nonverbal reactions as you step into his or her personal space.

Were you aware when your partner became uncomfortable? What signs did you observe in your partner that made you aware that they were experiencing you as too close? Go into as much detail as you can. This can include body posture, movements or stillness, skin color changes, eye contact or lack thereof, and a host of other behaviors.

Cautions about personal space

- DO NOT knowingly step into your patients' sense of safety or comfort, particularly during stressful times.
- DO NOT allow another person to trespass within your personal space, thereby accommodating them at the expense of your own sense of safety or comfort. It is important to be very conscious of your own physical sensations, thereby being able to define limits. For example, let us imagine that a patient moves into your space. You should say something like, "I am very interested in what you are saying, but you are standing too close to me. Move back about four feet and we can continue to talk." Such a firm statement is, in fact, an assessment tool. There is no better way to assess an individual's intention toward you than observing how he or she responds when you establish a boundary that you have a perfect right to set. You are dealing with very different individuals: when told to step or move a chair back, one may respond with profuse apologies and general nervousness; another may smirk and say, "What's the matter – are you nervous around men?"
- On other occasions, particularly with youth, you can set the limit humorously. "Jeez, Allie, you are just about standing in my pockets. Give me a little room to breathe here!" Be careful that the patient does not misinterpret your humorous limit setting as making fun of them or not taking them seriously.

Becoming Mindful of What You Already Know

Carry a small notebook with you for one week. When you interact with someone who is sad, depressed, angry, manipulative, friendly, loving, and so on, pay attention to your need for more or less space and to your physical sensations. Jot those down in your notebook.

Pay attention to subtleties. For example, you might find that you react differently to a man who is depressed than to a woman with the same symptoms. Through this, you will begin to learn to use your body to ascertain another person's moods or intentions – that when, for example, someone is angry, you feel a tightness in your neck, whereas when a person is sad, you feel a desire to move away from them.

Some of your physical reactions may be unpleasant or unflattering to your own self-image. For example, let us imagine that you get somewhat sick to your stomach when facing an aggressive person, or experience a subtle but real sense of revulsion when dealing with someone who is depressed. As unpleasant as some of these reactions may be, you do not need to change them. In fact, they are a treasure. You are neither your feelings nor your emotions. These are experiences that occur within you, but you do not need to identify yourself *as* them. Instead, you remain aware of your core sense of self – your integrity. When you are a person of integrity, your feelings and emotions convey information, even an urge to act in a certain way, but they do not *require* that you act.

If you continue to hone your awareness in this matter, you will develop a form of intuition called **MINDFULNESS**. Mindfulness is the ability to be consciously aware of what is going on in your interactions with another person.

Think of how being mindful will help you in your relationships with your patients. You will readily pick up on their level of discomfort. You will also begin to perceive the things you do that, despite your good intentions, appear to aggravate or frighten them. The texture of relationship is an increasingly nuanced understanding of other people's moods, NOT just the mentally ill individuals you encounter in your work.

Who is more dangerous?

Let us imagine two individuals, both of whom served time in prison for a life-threatening assault on another person. The first smirks and describes how he fractured the skull of a rival drug dealer. He airily says that he'd never do anything like that again, "because I'm not in the business anymore." The second describes, in a tone of outrage, how he went to a club with his wife, and while he went to pick up their drinks, returned to find a man mauling her sexually. He broke a glass and slashed the man's face, blinding him. Which man is more dangerous? <u>We don't know</u>. We do know, however, that the context of their aggression is poles apart. Furthermore, they tell their stories in very different ways. One obviously savors the opportunity to recount his violence and probably savored the act as well. The other is horrified by what he did but still feels justified in doing it. Their triggers are different, which suggests that they need quite different case plans and interventions, were either of them to become enraged.

Intuition: That small voice that you must respect

There must be free communication of and respect for each other's intuitions. Such gut feelings are sometimes tenuous, sometimes vague, but often the *first* signs that you are in a dangerous situation.

- People, embarrassed, often minimize such intuitions as they inform others about their concerns, saying, for example, "I know it's nothing, but . . ." In doing so, they inadvertently lead others to minimize the situation.

- Others will muse, "He seems like the kind of guy who you read about in the paper with four bodies buried in the back yard . . . Jeez, where did that thought come from?"

- Some people inadvertently cloak their concerns through black humor or jokes: "Watch out, she's going to come back tomorrow and go postal." In saying this in an offhand manner, one tries to avoid the sense of fear that one really feels. In joking about it, however, one can easily convince both oneself and others that the concern is not valid.

- People do not voice their hunches at all, feeling awkward or embarrassed because they do not have "hard evidence."

- Others are inhibited by pseudo-ethics such as "not stigmatizing the patient," or believing that others will view them as some "ist" (racist, sexist, homophobic) if they have a negative intuition about someone from a designated oppressed or outcast group. For example, a young man from a certain ethnic or lifestyle group (take your pick) is vaguely threatening toward staff – but the agency itself has already become divided by "identity" politics. A staff person voices some concern about him but is immediately jumped on because "you are just making that assumption because he's _____."

- "Logical" individuals or senior members of staff, sometimes those who *claim* to have the most experience, are the ones who belittle others' intuitions of danger.

Differences among staff must be discussed respectfully, particularly when they involve questions of safety. In many circumstances, each person has only part of the picture. If one person's idea or intuition is discounted or dismissed out of hand, he or she may cease to speak up – and vital information regarding everyone's safety is lost.

Example: Lifesaving intuition

Visiting a home for a mental health evaluation, I sensed something inside me, very powerfully, that ordered me not to knock on the door and to retreat to my car. I wrote in the homeowner's new chart (she had been referred by her concerned landlord) in huge red letters, "Something is wrong. Do not go to this house without police backup." As unprofessional as my supervisor deemed this note, it had to remain in the chart, as state law required that no chart note be destroyed. Thankfully, a coworker heeded my "irrational" advice, and several days later, she and the police found a floridly psychotic woman waiting behind the door with a gun. In a previous psychotic episode, while in an isolated area in the Alaskan bush, she had been attacked by two men intent on raping and murdering her. She held them off with a gun and was eventually rescued by police. Now, some years later and again in a psychotic, very paranoid state, she was waiting with her gun, having seen me approach the house. It is probable that only my <u>not</u> knocking on the door saved my life. When my coworker went to the house with her rescuers – because that is how the woman viewed police – she willingly turned over the gun. What did I perceive? Was it a stirring of the curtains, a soft click of the bolt of an automatic weapon being pulled back, or ESP? To be honest, I don't care. What matters is that I – and anyone I work with – respect such intuitive commands.

An Early Warning System

Beyond the ability to more accurately perceive what another person is feeling, this practice will give you the ability to anticipate people's intentions. It is one thing to be aware of the hollow feeling in the pit of your stomach when someone stares at you hostilely across the room. It is another to recognize your experiencing that same discomfort when a patient says something ostensibly benign, where <u>if you have the same reaction you have when someone is threatening you, it is very likely that this smiling patient means you harm</u>.

Example: The need for an early warning system

A patient once said to me upon termination of services, "Thank you. No one has ever treated me with respect like you did before. It's hard to think that I must stop seeing you. You've helped me so much." Despite his gentle voice and smiling face, I had the very powerful reaction that I always have when someone overtly threatens me. However, young at my trade, I brushed off the warning, thinking, "I am being silly – the man just complimented me." Sometime later, he poisoned me. I am only alive today because he chose to degrade me by contaminating my food rather than putting something lethal in it. I learned in the bitterest way possible to always pay attention to what my body "tells" me. <u>The body is linked to the most primitive areas of the brain, structures that serve to protect us from danger through pattern recognition rather than verbal cognitions</u>. To treat our bodily reactions with disrespect is to disavow that which has kept humanity alive for eons.

CHAPTER 27

A Fair Witness

There may be nothing worse than feeling helpless or shamed after experiencing a physical or emotional attack. This is especially the case when a patient – someone for whom you are, to some degree, responsible, and to whom you have pledged help – is aggressive or even violent toward you. One often feels terribly alone when under assault, even with others present. This sense of isolation gets far worse if there is no one to talk to about it.

Those who work in hospitals and other care facilities have a particular dilemma because we are bound by rules of confidentiality. Furthermore, some of the things that affect us most are so ugly or appalling that, were we to bring it home to discuss in detail with a mate or other family member, we would, in effect, be inviting violence or obscenity into our homes. It is sometimes a mark of courage and decency to forebear passing the burden of grief or horror on to a loved one. Therefore, many of us must cultivate peer support. This can include strategizing sessions or co-supervision, but there are times when this is the last thing we need. Instead, we simply need someone to demonstrate by their presence that they, too, share this dilemma: that there are times when we cannot help, and other times when it is those to whom we offer the best of ourselves who threaten or hate us the most.

In such circumstances, we need fair witnesses, people who share the same type of work, who know you, who respect you, and who are willing to hear you out. These are people to whom you can speak about what you have gone through, and who are strong enough to stand in the face of your pain or outrage. They are not there to solve your problem or to coach you. A fair witness informs you, often simply by their presence, that you are still a part of the human family, a valued member of your hospital, despite the isolation you may feel as a result of the terrible situation you have experienced.

SECTION V

Suicide

CHAPTER 28

Core Components for Assessment and Intervention with Suicidal Patients

It is difficult for many people, even health care professionals, to believe that life's problems could be so terrible that suicide is even a consideration. For the suicidal person, however, it is an answer to the seemingly unending pain, trauma, and frustrations of life. They feel trapped, unable to conceive of an end to their torment, whether it is due to the actions of other people, or something generated from within.

Problem-solving activity that it may be, suicide is also an act of violence resulting in the death of a human being. That it is done by one's own hand does not make it any less murderous. This is a particularly important consideration because, given that there is hatred and often a weapon, your hospital must also consider the safety of other patients or staff who might have any connection with – or merely proximity to – the suicidal person. In short, the difference between murder and suicide is often nothing more than what direction the weapon is pointing.

The dangers within

Hospitals frequently do a very poor job of screening suicidal and potentially violent patients – particularly during the admission process in the ER. They are often placed in a treatment room, sometimes waiting for hours, with a variety of potentially lethal medications and sharps within reach. In many cases, they are placed in a secure room only *after* an interview with a hospital social worker that may have taken place many hours after their arrival. It is imperative that your hospital review admission procedures and consider if there are safer alternatives to leaving such volatile patients in an environment that is dangerous both to themselves and to hospital staff. See Appendix III for more details.

Warning Signs

Many books and training manuals on suicide focus on demographics, presenting lists that enumerate the suicide rates based on people's ethnicity, age, educational and economic status, traumatic life events, and so forth. Although such general information can be helpful, you need to notice what is significant about the individual patient, and not merely to which category he or she conforms. Nonetheless, there are some important warning signs that indicate that a person may be contemplating killing himself or herself.

- Significant negative changes in your patient's life, such as divorce or a romantic break-up, the death of a loved one, victimization such as abuse or violence, events such as conflict or fights at school or the worksite, any humiliating incident or disappointment such as being dropped from a team or club in the case of youth, or the loss of employment in the case of an adult.

- Other warning signs may include a radical change in clothing or appearance, particularly styles that set one apart from the society of which they were previously a member; hostility toward peers, workmates, family, or hospital staff; social withdrawal and isolation; the giving away of prize possessions; writings or drawings with morbid or despairing themes; a depressed demeanor; and allusions to a lack of a future or to the pointlessness of "it all," or, paradoxically, a sudden elevation in mood on the part of a previously depressed patient, which suggests the possibility that they've finally found a "solution" to their problem.

- The intangibles: Sometimes, without knowing why, you or another staff person has a sense of foreboding, or at other times, you think something "ridiculous," such as "I don't think that kid will live to see twenty," or "I wonder if this is the last time I will see this patient." Such thoughts are often – <u>very often</u> – an intuitive sense that something is very wrong. Approaching someone out of concern when your "evidence" is so vague requires some tact – but approach you must.

Approaching Intervention

To begin, you must ask yourself if you are the proper person to ask this patient any questions at all. Your hospital must have a very clear policy on how to respond to suicidal patients. It may be that your *only* responsibility is to speak to a designated person(s) who will take over the intervention with the patient. In this case, your task is to clearly organize what you have observed so that your concerns are considered with the gravity that they deserve.

Beyond one's specific responsibilities, this is not the place for grandiosity, where you think that because you are "good with patients," that this boy or girl, man or woman will open up to you. Do you *know* that this person respects you? Have you acted in ways that would lead them to feel otherwise? Have you been unsuccessful in establishing a relationship of trust with them, despite making a valiant attempt toward that end? To be sure, there are people who are isolated and alienated, and it is *only* through asking questions of concern that respect between you will be born, but you must at least have a sense that he or she does not hold you in either personal contempt or indifference.

If, however, you are the person who should speak with the patient, what must you do?

Where should you speak? Try to speak where you will have no interruptions. At the same time, you do not want a place that is so private that you and the patient are isolated. Remember, suicide is an act of violence, and in many cases, not just "harm to self."

Approach with the correct demeanor. Too much direct eye contact, close physical proximity, or an overly gentle, "concerned" voice may shut the patient down. Sit easily, but not overly confidently. If you present yourself as too "together," they may experience this as an implicit judgment on them, their lack of ease contrasting so dramatically with your confident demeanor. Consider sitting at an angle or even side-by side, with only an occasional glance toward the person. Eye contact, when it happens, will then have significance, rather than it being experienced as a constant, intrusive examination.

Meander. With wary individuals, you may wish to "wander around," so to speak, talking about this and that. Try to establish a dialogue, a connection with the patient, before asking the hard questions.

Do not be too "nondirective." Many people find "counselor's style," where the intervener only does "active listening" and "reflection," to be maddening. They must know who you are before they can trust you.[14] In establishing a dialogue, you are, of course, to maintain proper professional boundaries, but without conversation, there will be no contact between you.

Ask direct questions. When you have a real concern that a patient is considering or planning suicide, you must be more direct. Do not tiptoe around the subject, as vague statements leave the person an "out." The following would be an example of this mistake (the individual's inner thoughts are in parentheses):

Case manager: "Are you thinking of hurting yourself?"

Patient: "No, I'm not." *("Soon I'll be feeling no pain.")*

When a true concern about suicide arises, the correct question is, "Are you thinking of killing yourself?" Such a direct question often comes as a relief to suicidal people because it indicates that, at last, there is someone who is strong enough to listen to what is really going on inside them. If the person is not suicidal, they will let you know. If they are outraged by your questions, explain why you are asking them about the possibility that they intend to kill themselves. They should be able to give you a clear explanation why you do not need to be concerned. One final point: asking them if they have thoughts of suicide will not put the idea in their head if it was not there to begin with.

A failure to ask the right questions can lead to tragedy

How can a depressed or angry suicidal person trust you when you do not clearly state what the problem is? You might feel that this doesn't apply to you, but imagine a conversation with a weeping thirteen-year-old boy who tells you how scared he is because when his father comes home, he's going to be mad, because he took some money from his wallet. Of course, you ask if his father is going to hurt him. And the boy says, "No. He's never hit me. He'll just tell me I did wrong." You perhaps feel sorry for the boy, but you also think that maybe he'll learn a good lesson and not steal money from his dad to buy a video game. The problem is that you didn't talk long enough. You didn't hear the utter despair in his voice. You didn't learn what he means when he says that the father will tell him he did wrong. You didn't even think of suicide. If you had followed up with the proper questions, you would learn that the father will essentially flay the kid with his tongue, letting him know how useless he is, and how he wishes he'd had enough sense to have gotten his mom to abort him. Or, the father is not a bad guy at all, but this is a very sensitive kid: one of his friends killed himself six months ago, so the idea of suicide seems right to him, because then he won't have to face his dad, whom he let down so grievously in his own mind.

Speak in a calm, matter-of-fact tone of voice. If you sound nervous, you'll appear unreliable. If you're joking or off-hand, the patient will feel that you are not taking them seriously. If you are overly concerned, overly warm or "sensitive," you'll sound like a hovering counselor, that soft-voice, earth-tone-wearing, gentle soul who cannot be trusted to stand up and fight, but seeks refuge only in being "nice." If you are too concerned that you will overwhelm the patient with your energy, they will experience you as treating them as a) spun glass or b) playing games with them by trying to get them to reveal themselves while you do not. A calm, matter-of-fact tone shows that you are not panicked by their situation and that you can handle anything they can say. Remember it's their crisis, not yours. Your job is not to save them but rather to offer them all the resources and strength you can so they can save themselves.

No matter what the circumstances, you must have an attitude that you have all the time necessary to solve the situation.

- If you try to hurry things along, the patient will believe you are not actually concerned at all. And, instead of opening up and discussing their issues, they may very well "shut down" or simply give you answers that ease your fears.
- On the other hand, if you "buy" their sense of time, that a solution must be created right now, you too will act as if life-and-death must be decided in a matter of moments. Then there will be two of you in crisis.

When you take time, you give time – the patient begins to believe that there is enough time to figure out a better solution than suicide.

Don't give advice too soon. Until you become more familiar with the situation, don't hand out advice. Even then, keep it to a minimum. For example, if you immediately say, "Think of your family," the individual might mentally reply, "Yeah, they'll be sorry. Their tears dropping on my grave are the best payback I can think of!" The assessment process is a means to get them to reveal themselves and, therefore, feel less isolated. Furthermore, this gives you enough information so that you have some assurance that your interventions will not fall on deaf ears, or worse, support their drive toward death.

Never dare them to do it. That kind of stupidity only works in the movies. Do not belittle previous unsuccessful attempts as further proof of their failures, or as mere attention-seeking behaviors. The archetypal stupid sentence is, "Cutting? If you were serious, you would cut your wrists lengthwise, not cross-wise." "It's obvious," the aggressive intervener thinks, "that they are attention seeking and not serious," and he or she tries to shock them with the reality of what they are doing. Typically, such "interventions" are born out of frustration, irritation, burnout, or plain dislike of the often repeatedly suicidal person. It is a statement for us, not for them.

Don't get in a debate, particularly a religious debate. Some people use suicidal behavior as a way to feel some personal power in a world over which they have little control. Debates about the meaning of life, the nature of heaven, or the immorality of suicide will break rapport, and will likely aggravate one or both of you.

Use the power of dialogue. The most powerful intervention with suicidal individuals is that you are talking. The suicidal person, almost invariably, feels completely isolated, cut off from life and from people. A sustained, respectful conversation conveys on an almost primal level that they are still worth something, because you, who are worth something, finds them worthwhile to speak with. Communication itself heals.

CHAPTER 29

The Essential Questions
to Ask the Possibly
Suicidal Person

The following are the standard questions for assessing suicide risk. As you can see, there is a progression in which greater specificity indicates greater danger. You may not be a therapist, but even if you were, the basic questions would be the same. If not a professional trained in suicide intervention, you are assessing if the patient is safe or not and then determining if you need to contact the hospital social worker, the therapist or psychiatrist, parents, a spouse or partner, other caregivers, a mental heath professional, or the police. If you have a direct role in intervening with suicidal patients, you will continue with crisis intervention strategies once the basic questions are answered.

As always, your tone should be calm, straightforward, and nonthreatening. Do not use the following questions as a mere "checklist." Instead, use them in the natural flow of the conversation while understanding that the individual may wander off on all sorts of tangents before being ready to answer the next question.

The Four Questions
Question 1: "Are you planning to kill yourself?" If they answer no, follow up with questions and statements why you believe they might (e.g., "Your boyfriend called and stated that you told him that you were going out in a blaze of glory tonight. And then you said, 'Don't look for the body.'"). If they cannot adequately allay your concerns, then you may need to call emergency response personnel to assure their safety despite their denials.

If the patient replies something along the lines of, "I don't want to kill myself, but sometimes I pray that I won't get up in the morning," this could be termed passive or soft suicidal ideation. Do not minimize this, as the person's pain is very real although their lack of an immediate plan usually allows you sufficient time to refer these patients for a mental health intervention or further consultation with other members of their treatment team.

If the patient simply refuses to answer (e.g., "I'm not telling you that" or "You'd stop me if I told you that"), link them up with proper personnel for an assessment if you have collateral evidence that they might be suicidal. It should not be your job to cozen out the "maybes." We need to find out if they are playing games. If you are in a clinical role, then, with enough collateral information, you may insist that they be hospitalized, despite their refusal to answer any of your questions. **NOTE: The answer "I'm not telling you," at any point further in this process, should engender the same response.**

If the patient answers yes, that is a clear sign of their thought processes and intent. Depending on your role, follow up this answer with more detailed questioning, or take immediate action to ensure the patient's safety.

Question 2: "How would you do it?" Obviously, you will ask this question if the patient answers yes to question one. If their response is "I don't know," then you usually have time to address the issue by negotiating an agreement to seek or accept treatment after further supportive discussion. You have to find out if there are any impediments to seeking treatment, such as, "My dad would kill me. He hates counselors and says he's not going to waste any money on me." Or, "I'm not going to see a counselor. All they do is look at you and repeat what you say."

If the patient says that they "could do it all sorts of ways," offering a long list of possibilities, or simply says, "I'm not telling you that," this is manipulation. This does not mean they won't make an attempt, but their response usually stems more from an "I'll show you!" attitude. At this point, you must make it clear that such suicidal threats are taken seriously. Have them taken into custody or evaluated by a mental health professional rather than dancing around, so to speak, trying to coerce from them how serious they really are.

If the patient specifies a particular method (poison, overdose, hanging) or weapon (firearms or edged weapons), the level of risk has just increased exponentially. Sometimes, the suicidal patient will offer a plan and a backup plan – for example, "I want to jump off a bridge, but I think I don't have the guts. So, if I can't, I'll just OD." This is equally serious to a single method, because it denotes careful planning.

Question 3: "Do you have the means to do it?" Suicidal people may have decided on a method, but it is one that they have not yet acquired or have access to. Be sure to ask follow-up questions to ascertain if they have access to the method they've named. If they name a weapon, this immediately becomes a security issue, if you do not know whether they have it in their possession.

If there is any menace or provocation in their demeanor while mentioning that their method of suicide is a gun or a knife, expeditiously separate yourself from the patient and call police. On other occasions, you can simply ask if they have the gun or the knife on their person. If they reply in the affirmative, remove yourself from their presence and call police. Do not ask them to give it to you for safekeeping: they may change their mind in the middle of the action and begin to struggle with you for possession of the weapon.

Example: Possible dialogue around possession of a weapon
(NOTE: There are many possible scenarios: this example is offered to show a case manager who demonstrates calm and the ability to think on their feet.)

Patient: "I want to shoot myself."

Case manager: "Do you have a gun?"

Patient: "I have it in my coat pocket, right here."

Case manager (**although surely frightened, remaining calm in demeanor**): "Louis, I'm going to get up and leave now. You know that hospital policy prohibits bringing weapons on site, and I'm going to call for someone who can put that in safekeeping for you."

Patient: "I won't shoot myself here. Listen, I'll give the gun to you."

Case manager: "I don't know anything about guns. And furthermore, I don't have the authority to do that. So, here's what we will do. I'll go out and call someone who can put the gun in safekeeping for you. <u>After</u> I step out of the room, I want you to put the gun on the floor over there – yes, right there, where it can be seen from the door – and then you return to your seat and wait for that person to come."

At this point the case manager gets up, leaves the room, and initiates procedures to call the police and to clear the area and/or go into lockdown, depending on the type of building.

Question 4: "When will you do it?" This question helps you to gauge immediacy and to determine if the patient has established the plan to make others suffer, and if there is anyone else who is "timed" to suffer (e.g. "on my mom's birthday").

The more "positive" answers you get to these questions, the greater the risk of a lethal outcome.

Follow-up Questions
In many cases, you will have fully accomplished all that you need to do. You know that the person is or is not suicidal, and how close to the act they are. In other situations, however, you may have to keep talking: perhaps they are beginning to trust you and want to talk more, or you are, in fact, the person responsible for clinical intervention. The following questions are designed to get more information and to keep them talking. As the patient continues to talk, they'll often pull back from the intent to kill themselves on their own, or they'll be more amenable to de-escalation because they feel that "at last,

someone is willing to listen to me." <u>Simple communication brings people away from suicide, even without a solution to the problems that drive a person toward it.</u>

- Sometimes, **AFTER** you have asked if they intend to kill themselves and they have denied such an intention, you can ask, as a follow-up, "Are you planning to hurt yourself?" Some people do not intend to die, but merely mutilate themselves. Again, this is a follow-up question: it should not replace the initial blunt question, "Do you intend to kill yourself?"
- "Have you tried to kill yourself before?"
- "Have you ever tried to do it another way?" Desperate people become very concrete and literal, only thinking of their chosen method. They may have made several attempts before, by other means.
- "Has anybody in your family or someone you cared about ever tried to kill themselves?" Such people have "shown the way."
- "Have you ever thought about suicide before this situation?"
- "How long have you been thinking about killing yourself?"
- "Have you been drinking? Using any drugs?" *(Don't push this one if you have a sense that the patient will be more worried about getting arrested for use or possession than finding a solution to the situation. In a hospital, of course, you have the wherewithal to do a tox screen, something to which most patients are not resistive.)*
- "What's happened that things are so bad that suicide makes sense?"
- "What else have you tried to do to get yourself out of this situation?" Be careful: a prickly person could respond by thinking or saying, "OH, SO YOU THINK I'M STUPID" or "NOW I HAVE TO EXPLAIN MYSELF AGAIN – I DON'T **KNOW** WHY HAVING A GIRLFRIEND AND STRAIGHT A'S ISN'T ENOUGH!"
- Other areas of concern include whether or not the individual has suffered any recent losses, is ill, or has little or no social or family support.

CHAPTER 30

The Art of Communication
with the Suicidal Person

Don't make guarantees of how wonderful life will be: rather, honestly explain the difficulties that lie ahead. For example, "No, I'm not guaranteeing counseling will help, and you will have to work hard in therapy; it won't be easy. In fact, it might be the hardest thing you've ever done, but it's something you haven't tried."

Don't be a cheerleader. If you are too active or too "positive," it will sound as if you think you are "in it together," thereby usurping their dilemma and making it your own. Paradoxically, when you act as if things are *too* important, the suicidal person begins to feel that they are doing things for you – not for themselves.

Don't try to bolster their "self esteem." You may be aware that they have talent, are attractive, or have a wonderful family. If you point this out to them – "You have so many reasons to live!" – you will most likely break rapport entirely. It is very likely that they know these things themselves. They look in the mirror and they see the beautiful face, but inside, they feel corrupt and foul. They look at their mom and dad, whom they painfully and deeply love, and think, "They would be so happy without me." They believe that their existence is an assault on their family. They have a talent – they know it – but even as they play the piano or basketball or do higher mathematics, all they feel is an aching misery.

Frame things with negatives to find out the trigger. "You've had a bad time – there is no doubt about that. Yet, somehow, you held it together all these weeks. What's different about today?"

Offer "revenge" through indifference. Sometimes a person will tell you a horrible tale of abuse or violation, particularly at the hands of their own family or someone else close to them, and now, all they want to do is die. Sometimes you can point out that their family's abuse was like a slow-motion murder, with this intention to suicide the logical outcome. Suggest that the sweetest revenge would be to be happy or indifferent to them. "It will 'kill' them. You will literally not care about them at all. Unlike now, they will have no ability to affect your life in the slightest."

> **Use caution**
>
> This use of the word "revenge" is not something you say at the beginning of such a conversation. You will usually note a tone of bitterness and anger – and you tap into this by suggesting that, through therapy, for example, the patient could learn to become indifferent to their abuser. "They will mean no more to you than dirt on the road."

Identify the intended "victims" beyond themselves. Try to ascertain whom the suicide is intended to hurt. You will be able, thus, to get a better sense if the patient is also homicidal, or on the cusp between self-harm and an intention to take other's along. We can tell if there are others intended to suffer when we ask:

- Who will find your body?
- Who will identify your body?

Some people are utterly shocked by these questions, so preoccupied with their own misery that they didn't even think that their children, for example, would be the ones to find them upon returning home from work. Others describe that same scene with happiness – hoping, thereby, that their family member will never have a good night's sleep again.

Don't wear your heart on your sleeve. Quite often the stories that suicidal people tell are heart-rending. However, this can also be a very sophisticated kind of manipulation. I am not trying to encourage cynicism here, but you must not allow yourself to become so emotionally involved that you feel betrayed, or simply burned out, if the patient rejects or minimizes your efforts to help. Ironically, contempt, irritation, or frustration are exactly what such patients expect from people, yet that is what their behavior elicits. You know you have lost your ability to center yourself in the crisis situation if you experience any sense of betrayal or hurt when one of the following occurs:

- You believe you are making progress, that you have formed an emotional, even spiritual, link with them. Then they suddenly curse at you, or accuse you of talking down to them or not caring.
- Others suddenly minimize everything they've just said, stating that they didn't mean it after all, and they cannot understand what you are so concerned about.
- They kill themselves – after all you have done, after struggling so hard to extend a lifeline to them and they kill themselves. You tried your best and they are dead.

One of the occupational hazards of working with people who suffer is that not all those in pain are endearing: some people are, to be honest, quite unlikeable. Others do not even have the ability or resources to accept help when it is offered. It is the hallmark of a professional that you do not become burned out simply because some people either play games, or are playing on a different field than you thought. Remember, they don't live for you. Therefore, do your best – and do it cleanly. Even if the other person turns out to be manipulative, abusive, or indifferent to your attempt to help them, ensure that you do your job with integrity.

Internal Questions that Sidetrack Us

- "I don't know if I would want to live in such a miserable situation." It's not about you! The fact that they are talking with you means they still have some hope for another answer. Remember, dialogue itself here. Sometimes all they are asking for is a fair witness (Chapter 27).

- "Why is it important that they live?" or "I know I should care, but I don't." In cases like these, make death itself your enemy. The individual contacted you: your attitude should be that you will do your level best to speak for life. Not by evangelizing based on some spiritual belief, but simply in speaking in strong, calm tones, you are, in effect, a voice from the land of the living to one trying to cross over into the land of the dead. ***Not on your watch!*** If they wanted to die, they shouldn't have come into contact with you!

CHAPTER 31

Suicide as Self-murder:
A Taxonomy

This is a tool that can be used to help gauge the seriousness of the person's suicidal intent, and what type of suicide it might be. In many ways, it is an amplification of the question, "Who is intended to suffer the suicide?" We ask these questions so that we can best work with the person, or pass them on to whoever will continue the intervention beyond us. Given that suicide is a form of murder – that of oneself – let us categorize it by roughly the same subdivisions that we do homicide.

- **Aggravated 1st degree self-murder**. This would include killing oneself in a heinous or torturous way, drinking acid or lye, for example, because the person believes he deserves to suffer. Another example would be a suicide calculated so that a loved one will find the body. A third would be a murder-suicide: killing oneself after killing family members or other people.

- **Premeditated 1st degree self-murder**. This would include any planned suicide. The majority of the people whom you speak with will fall into this category – that is why the standard assessment questions are concerned with planning.

- **2nd degree self-murder**. This includes impulsive actions that are usually due to extreme emotion or intoxication. It is rare that you will be on-scene in an event like this: it is unlikely that a person would go into an explosive personal crisis in the hospital itself. It is, however, more common in assisted-living environments. For example, a young woman breaks up with a guy in front of their friends, and he is so humiliated that he ends up on the roof threatening to jump.

- **Assaultive self-harm with intent to commit mayhem (1st degree self-assault)**. In this case, the person doesn't necessarily intend to die, but they do something horrible to themselves, often with the intent to show others how much they are suffering.

Example: Assaultive self-harm with intent to commit mayhem

A young man, just released from foster care at age eighteen and now living with his father, returned home to find his father on the couch having sex with the young man's new girlfriend. (He was unaware that his girlfriend shared affection for crack cocaine, his father's drug of choice.) The young man pulled out a fish boning knife and stabbed himself right in the abdomen. Miraculously, the flexible blade threaded its way between his internal organs, and all he needed was a few stitches. He said to me, "I didn't want to die. I didn't even think of that. It's just that my dad has always done stuff like this to me. Every time I trust him, this is the result. I guess I didn't know whether to stab him for doing it, or stab me for being stupid enough to trust him again."

- **Assaultive self-harm**. This includes more minor suicidal gestures, cutting on oneself and other self-mutilating actions (Chapter 32).
- **Self-sacrifice**. Rare though it may be, this includes actions that have the intention of helping others – like throwing oneself on a grenade to save one's comrades.

Example: Self-sacrificial suicide attempt

A young girl, aged twelve, was being sexually abused by her father. She suffered it for years, but her mother slapped her in the face for "talking dirty." When her father began turning his attention to her younger sister, she thought, in the irrational magical way of a child, that if she did something as awful as suicide, maybe someone would help her sister. Thankfully, her attempt to kill herself failed, and a very good hospital social worker asked her the right questions, thereby getting help for both girls.

- **Self-execution**. This includes suicide that is primarily directed by a sense of guilt at things that should be morally condemned. (Many suicidal people feel guilty. This category is confined to those who have actually done some severe transgression and the only expiation they can think of entails their "execution.")
- **Mercy self-killing**. This category includes so-called "assisted suicide" or other suicides in which the person is seriously ill and wishes to "die with dignity."
- **"I'm taking my body out of here."** This is an attempt at final control over one's fate, something that can range from an act of heroism against intolerable violation or oppression to the act of a psychopath in prison whose only way of thwarting the people who hold him against his will is to kill himself.
- **Survivor's guilt**. This is a terrible outcome of good fortune, something we see all too frequently among soldiers who have survived combat while their comrades have not.

Take note of the type of suicide the patient is moving toward. This will help you or those who take over the case to know what direction to move with them.

CHAPTER 32

Self-mutilation

One of the most confusing actions that a person can do – at least to those outside the situation – is self-mutilation. When it is an enactment of something that looks like a suicide attempt, but somehow has survival "built in," it is referred to as "parasuicidal behavior" (Chapter 33). Here are examples of self-mutilating behaviors without suicidal intent:

- Rubbing an eraser on the wrist until all the skin is peeled away and one has a weeping lesion in the flesh.
- Repetitively stubbing out a burning cigarette on one's face and genitals.
- Running a needle in and out of the flesh of one's belly.
- Hacking open one's wrists on the corner of a table, and then, after being stitched up, tearing out the stitches with one's teeth and attempting to spray blood on nearby hospital staff.
- *Compulsive* rather than cosmetic body adornment, particularly that which is transgressive and outside of social norms.
- Slicing open the abdominal wall all the way to the fascia that holds the organs.

The hallmark of all of these actions is that the person does not intend to die. Even in the last horrifying example, the woman in question, a former nurse who uses a scalpel with the skill of a surgeon, calls for help after she makes the cut.

There are a number of reasons why someone would do such acts:

Self-hatred. The individual punishes himself or herself through self-torture and disfiguration.

Attention seeking. These cases usually, but not always, are typified by more superficial wounds. Such individuals "require" others to pay attention to them, particularly family members or loved ones who become afraid that they will be responsible for their death if they do not act. In the case, cited above, of the young man who threaded a needle in-and-out of the folds of his belly, he was an unpopular, socially inept boy who craved attention. By means of this action, he received some; in fact, at least once a day, other students at his school would dare him to do it again.

"Primitive medicine." Similar to the historical European and American medical practice of bloodletting to "cure" a variety of physical and mental health illnesses, these patients are metaphorically "draining out" the poisons in their bodies by bleeding themselves.

A struggle to feel something. Some people, in the throes of deep depression or trauma, literally feel numb. Absent any apparent emotions, they use these torturous acts to help them feel alive.

Stress reduction. Physical wounding results in the release of endorphins, neurochemicals that have a pain-relieving effect similar to opiates such as morphine and heroin. A common example of this is the "runner's high" that people experience after a particularly vigorous workout. People can become habituated to endorphin release, and activities that stimulate it can become addictive. One cuts to feel a sense of well-being.

Example: Self-mutilation for the reduction of stress

A young woman told me, after years of verbal and emotional abuse by her father, "I felt like I was walking on egg shells all the time. Then, when my mom and I finally left, it was like I couldn't stand any emotions at all. Even when I was happy, I would still feel like I was going to explode." She described one day cutting herself on the forearm with an Exacto knife, and to her shock, feeling a sense of warmth and peace. Not psychological warmth alone, but a warm floating sensation as well. Several weeks later she tried it again, and soon, it became an addiction.

Rehearsal. Some patients want to commit suicide, or profess to do so, but their underlying fears make them hesitant, resulting in numerous "failed" attempts at suicide.

We must also recognize that the line of self-mutilation has "moved." We see individuals who have tattooed much of their body, or have multiple piercings, including their tongue or sexual organs, who have voluntarily branded themselves, and others who even have metal implants placed under the skin, to end up, for example, with "devil's horns." Most of these people talk about endorphin release. Many refer to themselves as "modern primitives," stating that they are making their own bodies into works of art.

Clinically, we should be concerned with the following types of individuals:
- One who manifests emotional stress or depression, or otherwise displays some of the warning signs enumerated in the previous chapters on suicide. This is, by definition, an emergency.
- Self-mutilation that is a sign of severe psychopathology, either due to a psychotic process or a terrible abuse of oneself. This requires triage: Is it an emergent situation? Do they need to be detained in a hospital because their psychosis may lead them to do irrevocable harm to themselves? Is this a manifestation of a severe character disorder, so that the person would benefit from a referral to a particular type of therapy best suited to help them with their situation?
- It is simply a medical emergency, where the person had no intention of harming him- or herself, at least as far as they are concerned. Imagine a person who has undertaken do-it-herself splitting of her tongue in emulation of a snake, something this author has seen. However, in this case, the bleeding doesn't stop and the wound is septic. Triage is based on risk, not aesthetics.

The best way to answer these questions is to ask some. Go through a standard assessment on suicide, if required, and beyond that, interview the person in enough depth so that you understand their intention in their self-mutilation. Through this process, you will make the best clinical decision about what kind of help, if any, that they need.

CHAPTER 33

Crying Wolf:
Identifying and Helping
Parasuicidal Individuals

You surely have some patients who seem to be in or seem to create a constant state of crisis. Everything is an issue, and the most minor problems or setbacks are likely to cause an inappropriate amount of emotional stress and drama. Such patients frequently resort to repeated suicide attempts or threats, or self-mutilating acts that we referred to in the last chapter as parasuicidal behaviors.

A hospital – even a psychiatric hospital – should NOT try to manage this type of behavior alone. Instead, you need to set up a team that includes outpatient professionals seasoned in dealing with parasuicidal individuals. The task of this team will be to devise a strategy that does not reward the behavior, while at the same time does not punish or ostracize the person. If we overly nurture the patient, or hover around them, however, this "negative attention" rewards the behavior that we want to forestall. Paradoxically, a good plan sometimes requires us to be firm and noncommittal, and to set very strict limits so that the patient has little or nothing to gain, at least from external sources, in making the parasuicidal action.

At the same time, one must cultivate an ability to emotionally reward any healthy behaviors, no matter how rare they are. Parasuicidal individuals usually have a limited ability to reward themselves. Emotional rewards must come from outside. We often ignore such troublesome people when they aren't acting out, because we feel that they already take up too much of our time. If we do not emotionally reward them during times when they are not creating crises, these people never experience anything good coming to them. When they begin to experience something good coming from acting good, then they begin to learn how to reward themselves.

Parasuicidal Behavior Is an Act of Violence against Society

All too often, our focus centers on the person enacting the pathology. Their acts affect many other people as well. Such repetitive parasuicidal actions are, however, whether the person intends it or not, acts of violence against the fabric of society. Let us consider the damage that results from their actions:

Compassion burnout. Quite simply, we get sick of such people. Despite our intentions to the contrary, we often see them only as manipulative, self-involved, pathetic losers. Beyond whatever justification one might create for that point of view, it unfortunately expands. Many professionals begin to view all suicidal people, at least those with personality disorders, through the distorted lens that burnout creates. This becomes a safety issue. When we begin to view others with contempt, they can easily respond with their own negative emotions. Thereafter, interactions between such patients and hospital staff become increasingly volatile. Remember, too, that a mentally ill, perhaps suicidal, patient might have a negative interaction with one contemptuous staff person and decide to take it out on another, at a later date.

Damage to society. Suicidal threats, alone, can take up an enormous amount of hours, not only for hospital staff, but also for law enforcement and the entire emergency medical system. With our economy severely stressed, and our medical system currently in unknown financial waters, the hundreds of thousands of dollars that may be needed, every year, to manage the behaviors of a single parasuicidal patient make such acts, from one perspective, acts of violence against our society. The bottom line is that hardworking citizens pay for any public service.

A Plan for Patients Who Make Repeated Suicidal Threats

A committee needs to be set up to figure out the best way to deal with the situation. Ideally, this committee should include representatives from law enforcement, parole/probation, emergency medical response, hospital ER, the mental health system, and the prosecutor's office.

If the person has made repeated suicidal threats without suicidal acts, resulting in repeated calls to 9-1-1 and emergency response from law enforcement and EMT, consider prosecution among your other options. Among the charges that can be levied are false reporting, abusing the 9-1-1 system, and interfering with medical care. While in detention, it is the responsibility of the mental health system to maintain contact with the person and begin to work with them so that they get a sense of reward when NOT using suicidal threats for attention.

Arrest and incarceration can be an act of compassion

Some professionals have reacted extremely negatively to this type of suggestion, which I have made frequently during consultations in various locales. I have been accused of a lack of compassion, of blaming the victim of mental illness. It is my position that mental disorders are as much social constructs as they are illnesses, particularly personality disorders such as borderline personality disorder.

I have been very much influenced by Japan's *Morita Therapy*, which postulates that one clear sign of mental illness is "selfishness," a relinquishing of a sense of responsibility toward others.

Those with personality disorders, in particular borderline personality, believe that their feelings are all important. Therefore, if they feel horrible, they are justified in misusing the emergency system. If we can assist such an individual in realizing the impact of their actions on others, that police and firefighters were not born to serve them, and that their actions cause their family profound pain – we are thereby helping them toward health.

I have seen single acts of prosecution for false reporting do wonders for people. How? All of a sudden, they realize that their acts have implications.

I am aware that this sounds very harsh, but if an individual spends two weeks or even a month in a jail cell, visited regularly by their case manager, with a dedicated plan on how to manage their emotional pain upon relief, they very likely will do better. Over and over again, I have seen such individuals cease their abuse of the 9-1-1 system. With police and fire no longer appearing at their door, and an end to the drama they elicit around parasuicidal actions, such people actually begin to focus on becoming more productive members of society.

In sum, in situations where other interventions do not work, and the person continues to threaten suicide (requiring the attention of police, EMT, and emergency rooms), such prosecution and incarceration can be the epitome of compassion.

A Plan for Patients Who Carry Out Repeated Parasuicidal Actions

If they have actually enacted suicidal gestures, even wrist scratching or taking a few pills, prosecution is highly unlikely.[15] The risks of a more serious suicidal attempt will be viewed as too high. However, a comprehensive plan can be set up so that the individual gets more emotional rewards and attention by NOT engaging in parasuicidal gestures. Such a plan must be individualized: in other words, it must fit both the patient and the resources you have to offer. Therefore, rather than mapping out a general plan, I have included an example in Appendix I.[16]

SECTION VI

Recognition of Patterns of Aggression

CHAPTER 34

The Nature of Aggression

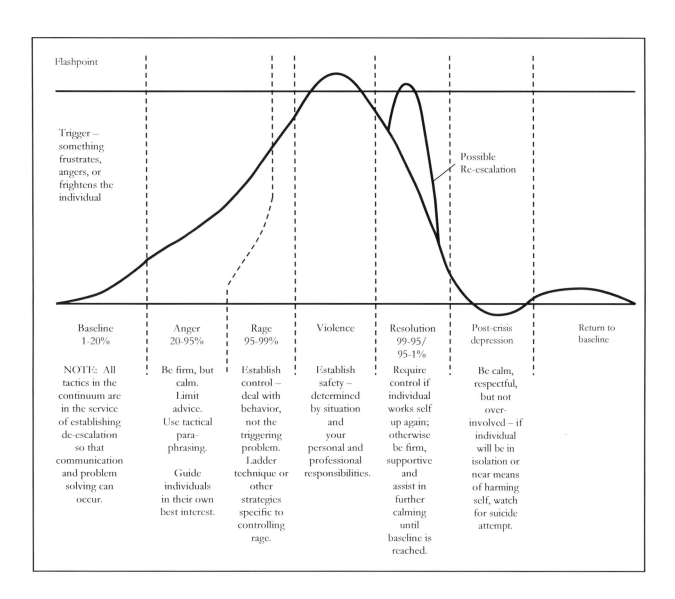

Baseline 1-20%	Anger 20-95%	Rage 95-99%	Violence	Resolution 99-95/ 95-1%	Post-crisis depression	Return to baseline
NOTE: All tactics in the continuum are in the service of establishing de-escalation so that communication and problem solving can occur.	Be firm, but calm. Limit advice. Use tactical para-phrasing. Guide individuals in their own best interest.	Establish control – deal with behavior, not the triggering problem. Ladder technique or other strategies specific to controlling rage.	Establish safety – determined by situation and your personal and professional responsibilities.	Require control if individual works self up again; otherwise be firm, supportive and assist in further calming until baseline is reached.	Be calm, respectful, but not over-involved – if individual will be in isolation or near means of harming self, watch for suicide attempt.	

The Cycle of Aggression

An outburst of aggression usually occurs in a cycle that starts with relative calm and ends with relative calm. The aggressive cycle usually appears to start with an apparent *triggering event*, though, in fact, the crisis may have been fulminating for some time. The reader may recognize the term "trigger," being familiar with it in terms of relapse in regard to substance abuse. The same concept applies with acts of violence. Just as many addicts have certain triggers that elicit the urge to use drugs, aggressive patients have triggers that cue them to become violent.

Baseline: from 0 to 20

When we are calm, we are at **baseline,** which is represented as 0 to 20 on the accompanying chart. At baseline, we use the parts of the brain most responsible for our finest human characteristics: thinking, creating, and forming social relationships. The rating scale goes up to 20, underscoring that one can have a little heat and energy and still be fully rational.

Anger: from 20 to 95

A triggering event elicits a change in both thinking and feeling. It can be something that threatens an individual's sense of safety, frustrates him because he hasn't gotten what he wanted, or simply cues him that he is now justified in using a skill (aggression) with which he is confident. Once aggression is triggered, the person becomes first irritable, then **angry**.

If baseline is presented as being 0 to 20 on the scale of aggression, with actual violence being 100, anger represents the numbers 20 through 95. If the person at baseline is eminently human, the angry person is the quintessential mammal. Regardless of the numeric value, the angry person is still trying to communicate with you. However, because we perceive their attempts to communicate as obnoxious, domineering, frightening, or irrational, we often do not construe their actions as communication. They, on the other hand, experience an increasing sense of frustration or even desperation at their inability to make themselves understood, further fueling their anger. Unfortunately, for many people with anger issues and poor coping skills, the bromide "if the only tool you have is a hammer, then every problem looks like a nail" applies. There are several reasons such people grow angrier as the perceived conflict continues:

- Some people simply cannot accept anyone disagreeing with them, especially when they believe they are right.
- When you do not seem to grasp what they are saying, you are perceived as being disinterested or too obtuse to understand.
- Your lack of comprehension implicitly accuses *them* of stupidity or unreasonableness.
- When you do not agree or comply with them, you are frustrating them in achieving something they desire.
- Many males have a misconstrued and hypersensitive sense of "respect," especially in the social context of our nation's inner cities.[17] Resistance, disagreement, or perceived slights are often seen as being disrespectful toward the person, causing them to lash out in anger or violence in an effort to regain their "street cred."

As people become more agitated, the areas of the brain that mediate basic emotions take over. At this point, equity, negotiation, or compromise becomes less and less attractive. In their increasing frustration, angry people attempt to dominate you: to *make* you either see things their way or simply comply with them, whether you agree or not. Their domineering behavior is, as much as anything else, an attempt to "get through" to you.

Think of arguments you have had when, frustrated, you said such things as, "No, that's not what I'm saying! Do I have to explain it again?" or "Let me put it another way!" or "You just don't get it! What do I have to say to make you understand?" We become progressively more intense, often raising our voices (as if that will help the other person understand) because we desperately want the other person to grasp what we are saying. This type of escalation is counter-productive, despite our intentions, because we tend to make less sense when we are angry.

Anger is accompanied by physical arousal that functions as a feedback loop, driving us toward further arousal. At this point, we no longer care about the truth: we care about being "right" and proving the other "wrong." The disagreement has become a win or lose situation. We interrupt more frequently, cutting other people off, and we only listen to pick out the flaws in their argument.

To de-escalate and control the angry person, you should attempt to "line up" with them, demonstrating that you comprehend what they are so intensely trying to say, thereby proving that their concerns are important to you too. ("Line-up" tactics will be the subject of Section VII.) This in itself is powerfully disarming, not only calming them down, but also helping you to work together to actually solve the problem.

Rage: from 95 to 99

How can we tell the difference between anger and rage? When someone is angry, you too may become angry. You might also become concerned, upset, hurt, confused, or frustrated. Usually, however, you are not afraid. Why? Although angry people may *later* become violent if they become further agitated, that is not their aim. Instead, their intention is to communicate with you, albeit dramatically, loudly, or forcefully. At worst they are trying to dominate or intimidate you so that you will do what they want. As abhorrent as this may be, it is still communication.

When people are enraged, however, they are, in effect, trying to "switch themselves on" to becoming violent. Many people slowly work themselves up, while others lash out violently with seemingly no prior warning, verbal or otherwise. Usually however, even uncommunicative patients will signal their anger or intentions through their body language and other nonverbal forms of communication. You should be aware of these warning signs of impending aggression, as manifested on the intuitive level (Chapter 26) and based on observable behaviors (discussed in the rest of this book).

Most of the time, anger does not result in violence. One reason for this is that people possess a number of self-inhibitors that work to control behaviors and prevent them from acting out their baser instincts. Within a state of rage, however, the person is *trying* to overcome those inhibiters, so that they can do what they actually desire: violence. What are some of the prime inhibitors?
- **A fear of consequences**. The fear of counterattack, legal consequences, social disapproval, financial costs, and a host of other possible negative outcomes serve to inhibit one's resorting to violence. This includes inhibitors that are innate to healthy neurological organization, as well as acquired inhibitors (for example, worrying about a loved one disapproving of what one desires to do).

- **Morality**. Although some political and social ideologies may define another group as less than human and, therefore, fair game for violence, most individuals possess a core set of moral principles that prevent them from harming others. It seems to be innate among most humans that, faced with the vulnerability of another human being, we find in their defenselessness a "demand" to treat them without violence.[18]
- **Self-image**. A man may see himself, for example, as the kind of person who does not hit women, make a public display of aggression, or lose control. A woman may see herself as caring, nurturing, and empathetic to the plight of the less fortunate. A positive self-image, and fears of tarnishing that image, will often preclude an individual from committing a violent act.
- **The relationship**. A feeling of responsibility toward the other person (e.g., friendship, love, and family relations) may hold an individual back from violence.
- **Learned helplessness**. Some people, survivors of abuse for example, have tried to defend themselves in the past and have failed repeatedly. They may believe that fighting back is a futile effort, only leading to further pain and abuse. Their rage, however, is there: inside. There are phrases like "a cornered rat" or "the worm turns," which describe a person who has suppressed their rage, sometimes for years, because fighting back always meant failure, pain, even destruction to them. Given enough frustration or threat, such people sometimes explode.

The enraged person, therefore, is simultaneously striving to overcome their self-inhibitors while another part of them struggles to maintain them. As their rage increases, they are no longer trying to communicate: they are working themselves up to an attack. Enraged people are like dinosaurs or lizards. Their rage is almost instinctive; they desire to destroy, not merely to become dominant.

What is the difference, then, between rage and violence? Anger is a rocket ship all fueled up with some fumes coming out, and the countdown initiated. Rage is right before liftoff. The rocket has not yet moved, but there are flames and steam billowing out, making a terrible roar, so loud the ground shakes. It is a roiling moment of explosive, tenuous equilibrium. Fuel could still be cut to the rocket engines so that it sits silent on the launching pad, but there are only a few moments to act, because the rocket is about to lift off. Liftoff is the equivalent of the initiation of **violence**.

What you *should* experience in the face of rage is fear. This is not a bad thing. Fear tells us that we are in danger and that we must do something – NOW! We will most likely be able to handle the situation, but we had better devote every power we have to survival. Fear demands attention, but it should not paralyze you into non-action, mentally or physically, in the face of anger and rage. Fear switches us on so that our internal emergency response systems are activated. A sense of powerlessness is a *conclusion* that some people reach when they are afraid, limiting their ability to control the situation or to defend themselves.[19]

Fear demands attention. A sense of powerlessness, on the other hand, is a *conclusion* that some people believe when they are afraid. Imagine two people about to be hit with a fist. One feels a sense of helplessness, a crumbling inward. The other feels a sense of outrage and instantaneously knows that they will somehow win. They have an internal sense that even if their body is wounded, their spirit will never be overcome. Fear can and should be a call to arms, not a sign of defeat.

To work with the enraged person, you must establish *control*, especially if the person's behavior presents an immediate threat to you or others. Control tactics, whether verbal or physical, are geared to establish the conditions that make the aggressive person no longer dangerous (recognition of specific rage states and controls tactics will be described in Section IX).

The difference between anger and rage

Imagine someone hands you a huge plastic container. Through its translucent sides, you can see a dark, hairy shape, a Goliath Bird-Eater, the world's biggest spider. It rustles around; its weight shifts the container in your hands as if it were filled with mercury. Is it creepy? Sure it is. Is there any reason to be afraid? Not really. As long as the lid is firmly on the container, you are absolutely safe.

This is the equivalent of anger: internally, you say, "I hope the lid stays on that thing. I'd better be careful how I hold this."

Now, imagine your friend takes the container back, bends down, and to your surprise and horror, takes off the lid. The spider emerges onto the floor right next to your leg. It raises its front legs in threat display and opens and closes its ¾-inch fangs. There is something poisonous, hairy, and mean in the room, and it is not enclosed in any container! The spider is out of the box. This, metaphorically, is rage.

However, the fear that now arises within you does not mean that you are helpless. You can still step on the spider or jump up on a table. A belief that you are helpless near the spider is an interpretation, not a fact. Fear is simply the warning cry – the drums at the brink of battle – that demand that you *must* act right now.

Violence: 100 on the Scale

Violence does not begin when someone is hit or injured. It can be perpetrated simply through the infliction of fear of imminent danger and attack. Some of the legal terms for this are terroristic threats, harassment, and harassment by communication, stalking, and menacing. In short, a violent act occurs whenever there is good reason to believe that you or someone else is about to be hurt. If the person does not have a weapon, we are talking about someone who is at about three arm's length distance and further approaching in a menacing way.[20] If the person is violent and has a gun, all the person has to do is point it toward you at any distance. Even if the weapon is not pointing at you, it is still violence if the person verbally or even implicitly threatens you. It is also violent when a person has violated personal boundaries and refuses to retreat.

Your guiding principle is <u>SAFETY</u>: You do whatever is most effective to protect yourself and the people around you. Whenever you can, the best thing to do is to escape and get help. However, if you are responsible for the protection of others, such as small children or disabled patients who are under your care, or you are otherwise unable to leave, escape may be either impossible or endurable. **Safety is defined by what you must protect**. This includes yourself, other vulnerable people, and, as delineated in our laws defining permissible self-defense, even the aggressive patient – as best you can in the circumstances you are facing.

The right to defend yourself

I must underscore that in the event of an actual assault when escape is impossible, it is an absolute human right to fight back in protection of yourself and other potential victims. That the aggressor may also be a suffering individual does not abrogate this right. I hope that you will never face such a horrible situation. At the same time, it is necessary to be clear with yourself, on a mental and spiritual basis, that you are willing to act in defense of yourself and others. You must do this now. Trying to discover this within yourself once the assault is occurring is far too late. Remember that protecting yourself is not only a personal matter. You are protecting everyone who cares for you from the harm that they will suffer if you are maimed or killed.

Self-defense tactics are well beyond the scope of this book. Those interested should consult with recognized experts in the field to find a self-defense program suitable for your needs. The essential principle of self-defense, however, is simple:

Imagine a door with seven locks and no keys. You are locked behind the door, and all that is good in life – your family, your love, your dreams, your values, even your integrity and dignity – is secured on the other side of the door. How will you go through the door? The answer, of course, is any way you can – with tooth and nail, and any implement you can reach. A violent aggressor is that "door." You have a perfect right to be on the other side.

CHAPTER 35

Why Would Someone Become Aggressive?

Aggression is not an alien or unnatural emotion. Without a capacity for aggression, humanity would never have survived. Yet most aggression seems far apart from the basic activities of hunting or self-defense. Much of it is irrational, self-destructive, vicious, or cruel. Why would someone be swept by rage when it causes so much harm? Why would people be prepared to throw away a future, even a life, driven by emotions that they themselves might be horrified to have expressed even a few moments later?

As you know from your own experience, there are many reasons to become angry, or even enraged. We can better establish safety with an aggressive individual when we understand what has driven that person to anger.

Anger and rage can develop because people are confused or disorganized. They can't understand what is going on around them or "inside" them due to cognitive distortions or a chaotic situation (too much information for them to figure out). Among those who experience this confusion are those who are profoundly mentally ill, autistic, developmentally disabled, intoxicated, or simply overwhelmed by emotion or the incomprehensible situation in which they find themselves. Imagine walking in a forest and suddenly a huge spider web drops on you. You thrash and struggle with all your limbs trying to get free.

Some people feel helpless, enclosed, trapped, or beset with a myriad of seemingly unsolvable problems. This is often similar in effect to confusion or disorganization, but it is accompanied by a particular anguish. The individual usually perceives one person or entity as the agent of their situation, and they desperately fight to get free from either their influence or their oppression. This sense of desperation could be elicited by being physically stopped from leaving when a person wants to go, being socially or otherwise intimidated so that they believe that they cannot leave, or becoming enmeshed in an argument that gets worse and worse and continues to escalate. In the latter case, people feel unable to speak sensibly and make others understand their point of view. Arguments between intimates frequently evoke this type of anger or even rage, where whatever one person says is "checkmated" by a response by the other. Mental health professionals sometimes elicit this rage in people when they analyze and interpret the patient's every action in an intrusive manner.

> ### Example: An "analytic attack"
>
> "William, I know you think you were acting out of altruism, but what you don't understand is that the reason you tried to help Joyce in the group is that she reminds you of your aunt. Your aunt was abused by her husband, and you had to stand by and accept it, being a little boy. When Joyce's nurse, Mr. Edmonton, appropriately set limits with her, you intervened, projecting the image of your abusive uncle onto him. Fortunately, no harm was done, but I am further concerned that you believe that, once again, you failed. You weren't able to stop what you incorrectly imagined was abusive."

The fear of attack elicited by perceived invasion of personal space is often a precursor to assault (Chapter 26). Particularly in stressful or volatile situations, you will be perceived as an attacker if you encroach upon another's personal space, no matter your intentions.

A demand for what they perceive as justice. It is rare that an angry person does not believe himself to be justified. Demands for justice are usually a complex sense of victimization or grievance and can include the following:

- The person feels that they are losing personal autonomy and power. The person feels dominated and oppressed, viewing themselves as fighting for their freedom. This sense of loss of power is personal; it doesn't have to be "true" in an objective sense.
- The person feels that their rights are either denied or being taken away. People who have a mental illness frequently have their freedom of action limited for their own safety, or to keep them from disturbing or interfering with other people. In such circumstances, many people experience a sense of violation when they are being limited or forced to conform to rules. Whether it truly is in their best interest or not, the person believes that something vitally their own is being stolen.
- A "self-appointed" revolutionary who is revolting against an unfair world, system, or group of people. The best sense of power that many people can achieve is in opposition to others. They welcome an opportunity to designate others as enemies, legitimate targets for their own animus. Such individuals, particularly those with paranoid ideas, believe that they and others are being oppressed by systems or powers beyond them. They are not fighting against interpersonal oppression, but against something they believe to be far larger; they "designate" you as a representative or exemplar of those larger forces.

Entitlement. For many people, entitlement is intertwined with desire. Their formula of life is that "if I want something, I deserve it, and if I am not getting it, I have a right to be more forceful in my demands so that it is given to me." Such a sense of entitlement justifies itself.

Hallucinations, particularly "command hallucinations." What drives aggression for some people is something "internal, yet external." The person is harried by alien voices that command them to do harm, the voice(s) asserting an all-powerful identity. The person may feel compelled to act as the voices demand, or become violent while trying to make the hallucinations stop. On other occasions, the voices, visions, smells, or sensations are simply distracting and irritating. Imagine your increasing annoyance with a mosquito whining in your ear, and when you try to hit it, all you do is hit yourself over and over again.

Material threats. People will fight to defend what they have or that which they believe they deserve. If a person believes that someone is intent on depriving him of his home, job, or possessions, violence can seem to be a logical choice. Any time involuntary hospitalization is considered, you must remember that you are thereby threatening the patient's living situation and employment.

Organic stressors including loss of sleep, insufficient or un-nutritious food, and fatigue. Brain chemistry changes when the human organism is stressed. This causes changes in perception, mood, and cognition, and among these changes can be an increase in irritability or hypersensitivity.

Recent stressors and losses. Anything that elicits profound emotion can cause the person to become volatile, and, hence, aggressive. This can include a recent death, a job loss, a divorce, an infidelity, or feelings of profound insecurity.

Intoxication. A "self-induced" delirium, intoxication leads to poor judgment. For other people, drugs and alcohol are not a "problem"; they are a solution. They drink or take drugs to "liberate" their violent desires, something frequently observed among perpetrators of domestic violence.

Ideology. Religious and cultural factors, be they the larger culture of a society, religion, or nationality or the smaller culture of a community or family, can provide an ideology that legitimizes aggression, even violence. Many cultures offer their members an "operating system" that expects a violent response in certain situations. Furthermore, cultures often define certain people or classes as inferior, even less than human. All too many cultures sanction violence against women as a matter of course. Any inpatient unit must be concerned about cultural issues. Contrary to any idea of political correctness, this must also include an education about the *pathologies* of particular cultures, and not just their positive aspects.[21]

Family interactions. One of the biggest motivators of aggression is what occurs within families. There is the friction of arguments regarding everything from house rules to who "owns" the house, the irritation due to living too close together, past grievances brought up with no resolution, and a host of other issues. An argument starts, but it quickly degenerates into a demand that each concede that the other is right. Each feels emotionally flooded and becomes more and more irrational, furious by their inability to "get through" to the other. This becomes all the worse when a family member is mentally ill because what they are arguing for may be irrational or delusional. Families often function as emotional traps – there is no escape from the people who, although loved, cause one the most pain.

> ### Where you live becomes your family
>
> Intensive case management, hospital wards, and residential treatment soon become family systems. Not only do patients and staff get involved in "transference relationships," where old family issues are replayed within the current situation, but the intimacy of the inpatient setting also becomes a family in its own right. It is imperative that supervisors of those involved in close or intense contact with patients include a consideration of what transference/counter-transference relationships are being created as well as the current "family-type" dynamics of the situation.

Romantic relationships. People in relationships often demand that the other person submit to their wishes. There are numerous grounds to fight, from money to sex to child care to infidelity. The rage is fueled by the same source: you will "love" me on my terms, even if the "relationship" is delusional, mere fantasy, or wishful thinking.

An individual who has already "given up." For some, aggression, like its mirror twin, suicide, is a "problem-solving" activity, a "what-the-hell" response when they cannot find any other solution. This is related to the person's belief that he has no effect on the world. Violence ensures that you will make an impact. Depressed people, particularly males, often manifest this type of aggression.

Shame/humiliation. One of the most powerful driving forces of aggression is a sense that one has been shamed. Shame is not a mild sense of social embarrassment; it is a sense of being exposed and victimized by others, with no hope of relief. Humiliation is a driving force for revenge-based aggression against staff, the patient reacting to something that they view, correctly or incorrectly, as causing them harm or offense. It is also a prime motivator for attacks when a patient has a transference reaction, identifying you with someone who shamed or violated them in the past. This type of reaction often smolders for a considerable time, until the person explodes into rage or violence, like an underground coal fire suddenly exposed to the air.

The Person Is Egged on by Others

- Some people are set up by others who are amused at getting them mad, a particular problem in inpatient psychiatric units where antisocial patients provoke others for fun.
- Other people are provoked by family members or friends who use the person as an instrument of their vicarious desire to inflict harm. For example, one patient hears from his father, "I thought you were more of a man. I can't believe you let that social worker talk to you like that." Or a teenager in an inpatient unit, who has been taunted over a period of time by other patients that she is a "suck-up" to the psychiatrist, proves them wrong when she suddenly assaults her doctor.
- Other people do this *to themselves* by "fronting," making a scene in front of others (friends or family, for example) to increase their status in their "pack." Then, out in front of everyone, they are afraid to back down. Others carry an "audience" inside their imagination. They require of

themselves that they conform to a fantasy of themselves as a fearsome individual whom others will avoid or submit to.

Violence as recreation. It may be difficult for some readers to accept, but for some people, hurting other people is perhaps the most pleasurable activity in their lives. There is a joy in making others submit, and for some, a delight in causing pain. If you attempt to deny this ugly truth, you will convince yourself that you are safe or in control and will remain for too long in the presence of such a dangerous person. Social services personnel sometimes work so hard at establishing what they believe is rapport that they do not realize that they have, figuratively, walked into a tiger's cage. Not everyone wants to be affirmed or validated. Some people revel in causing harm.

Surgical violence. This is a conscious tactic of intimidation. "I won't hurt you if you do X, but if you don't do what I say, I will hurt you very badly." This is criminal aggression, whatever diagnosis the person might have.

Protective rage. Not confined to parents, this is the rage expressed by one trying to protect another perceived as being victimized. The closer one feels to the victim, the more one's identity is "merged" with theirs, and the more fiercely aggressive the person will become. When we read a phrase that is associated with the kind of protection a parent has for a vulnerable child, we can fail to see that this, too, can be very dangerous. Not infrequently, one patient will intervene on behalf of another for what they believe are righteous reasons. For example, a patient throws something at a doctor and is physically escorted out of a common room in the ward. Another patient, in what he believes is chivalry, jumps on the back of a staff person because he believes the first patient was justified in throwing her pen at the psychiatrist.

Create an aggression profile

Look back at the list of reasons for aggression listed above and consider which applies to a particular patient. This information is most valuable in that it clarifies what preventive steps you can take and what strategies would work best for managing future aggressive behavior.

CHAPTER 36

Risk Assessment

Proper assessment of any patient entails a balanced mixture of objective and subjective data. Paradoxically, "objective" data is not objective until it has undergone a subjective review. You will pick up patterns that are not manifest in a cursory review of the lines on the page. Threat assessment must be qualitative, highlighting what is unique about each situation and each patient.

A Review of the Past

Take some time to reflect on the aggressive and/or violent incidents that have occurred among your patients. Looking over past incidents is a helpful and necessary first step in learning to manage crises more effectively the next time around. Here are the things to note:

- What were the circumstances that led to the aggressive incident?
- What was the *first* sign that the situation was getting volatile or dangerous?
- Remember what they said and what they did just before the incident started. Remember, too, the patient's body language prior to the incident.
- Consider what you thought and what you *physically* felt at each stage of the encounter. This may be the most important data you can recover. These sensations and emotions are the physical expression of intuition. When you next experience that same sensation, it is an early warning sign that a similar situation is developing (Chapter 26).
- What, if any, thoughts did you have to try to minimize, contextualize, reframe, or otherwise resist looking at the situation head on? In other words, did you make yourself unaware?
- What do you believe you should have done differently?
- What planning did you do in regard to that patient subsequent to the aggression? How happy are you with that plan?
- Did you report the encounter, and to what degree do you believe your agency backed you up? Staff must be encouraged to report any incident in which they felt threatened, even from a simple look or gesture. Over time, these reports will provide the data for a general representation of the more common threats that staff face when performing their duties. Safety protocols can then be fine tuned to concentrate on the most common threats, as needed.

Formal Threat Assessment Questions

Some agencies, particularly residential treatment facilities and mental health facilities, have rather extensive intake procedures. All too often, however, many agencies receive case files containing a bare minimum of information on the patient. Regardless of your agency's intake procedures and capabilities, obtain and review as much hard data about your patients (and prospective employees) as possible before scheduling them for a first office meeting.

The questions below are not an absolute predictor of aggression or violence. Nonetheless, if you are aware of the information below, you will have a much better idea who and what to watch out for. These questions also give you a basis for further, more detailed conversation to put the person's behavior in context. There is considerable overlap with the information in the last chapter. We are concerned, here, with a more objective enumeration of factors that may predispose someone to violence.

- **A past history of violence** is one of the most important factors in assessing risk. Violence is not only innate: it is also a learned behavior, which over time becomes easier to use as a problem-solving strategy. Furthermore, aggression is often quite rewarding to some people, who feel most powerful and in control when they are violent.

- **History of bullying or intimidation**. This is the psychological counterpart of physical violence.

- **Prior arrest**. Any arrest is a heightened risk factor, even if the arrest was for a nonviolent crime. The person may be terrified or outraged at the idea of being arrested again, or even having any more contact with law enforcement. They may view hospitalization as a form of incarceration. Furthermore, with the prevalence of assault, rape, and other forms of victimization within corrections institutions, the nonviolent arrestee may have come out a very different person than they went in.

- **Weapons**. In particular, we must be concerned when the person has a history of brandishing or using a weapon, talking about a weapon in menacing terms, or fantasizing in a pathological manner.

- **History of physical abuse or witnessing physical abuse and violence, particularly of a family member**. As with violence in general, domestic abuse is also a learned behavior. Some people, as children, bond with their abuser, and others simply develop a hair-trigger response to any sense that another person is trying to control, demean, or otherwise violate them.

- **Head injury or dementia**. Neurological injuries and afflictions are associated with impulse-control problems. Many of our young soldiers are coming home from 21st century combat with closed head injuries. Some proportion of them may have hair-trigger tempers and difficulty controlling negative emotions.

- **Fear of attack based on invasion of personal space**. Paranoid and fearful patients may lash out in defensive violence to any perceived threat. If you are properly "tracking" the patient, you should be aware if they become increasingly stressed with close physical proximity to you.

- **Poor impulse control and low frustration tolerance**. The inability or unwillingness to tolerate limit setting on their need for immediate gratification.

- **Recent stressors and losses**. Bereavement, separation, divorce, job loss, and other traumatic events can make one more willing to become violent. In some cases, the patient may feel as if he or she has nothing left to lose.

- **A feeling of victimization and grievance**. Some people may feel victimized by society in general or hold a grudge with "the system," in which their current predicament is always someone else's fault.

- **Drug and alcohol use**. Intoxicants act like solvents: they tend to dissolve the internal and social barriers that hold us back from our base desires, among them aggression. Of the many people whose violence is mostly associated with alcohol or drug use, one can say, "They don't have an alcohol (or drug) problem. They have an alcohol (or drug) answer. When they want to get violent, they know what to do."

- **Physical pain or discomfort (particularly chronic)**. This also includes the side effects of certain medications or withdrawal from drugs and alcohol.

- **The individual has already "given up."** Some people expect every interaction to be difficult or negative. Their pre-emptive response may be, "What the hell – nothing will help. If I'm aggressive, at least I can make my mark on the world . . . or on you."

- **Severe psychopathological symptoms**
  a. **Rapid mood swings**. Such people are unpredictable and can escalate into a rage unexpectedly.
  b. **Hallucinations, particularly command hallucinations**. When a person hears voices, the voices may be telling them to do something terrible. If you think someone is hearing voices, ask what they are hearing.
  c. **Mania** – a state of excitement, typified by rapid speech, grandiose thinking, very poor judgment, and impulsive behavior. People suffering from bipolar disorder (manic-depression) or intoxication on methamphetamine or cocaine may exhibit periods of manic behavior.
  d. **History of predatory or manipulative behaviors**.

- **Interactional factors between the aggressor and victim**. The aggressor views the victim as having power, being inflexible or controlling, or denying the aggressor his due. Such aggressors believe themselves to be the victim.

- **Religious and cultural clashes**. Staff should avoid any religious, political, or cultural debates with patients. However, staff should also make an attempt to be sensitive to the cultural mores and religious practices of their patients so they will not inadvertently insult them. By the same token, such cultural awareness should alert you to what, in the culture, sanctions violence against others.

Face-to-Face Interviewing

When a face-to-face interview is part of your threat assessment procedures, you may, depending on your professional role, address this using either a scheduled interview or a more free-form conversation in which the salient questions are seeded within a larger body of communication. As for the latter option, let us consider one concern as an example: disdain for authority. This can easily be observed without the interviewer ever having to ask, "Do you have the proper respect for those above you when placed in a hierarchical situation?" The patient or prospective employee often reveals his or her contempt right there in the room – sometimes directly to the interviewer. In other cases, when asked to describe interactions with people significant in their lives, they sometimes tell elaborate stories, complete with grievances and self-serving excuses, placing their happiness as the responsibility of others.

In many situations, you should flesh out any interviews with a record review and/or collateral interviews, speaking with others who are familiar with the individual. However, collateral interviews can present some logistic difficulties: confidentiality requirements may make it impossible for other professionals to communicate with you about your patients, and concerns regarding lawsuits around claims of defamation or libel may make other agencies unwilling to speak directly to you concerning prospective employees. Therefore, it is important that you are familiar with federal, state, and local laws regarding these issues.

Whenever interviewing a person of concern, ask direct questions about previous assault history and their potential for violence. Be sure to hold yourself in a calm, relaxed manner, offering a direct gaze, thereby communicating that you are asking for the information to better understand them, not because you are afraid. You are also trying to convey that you are able to handle anything they might mention, even angry or threatening statements. This can be accomplished through maintaining an air of quiet confidence and genuine interest in the patient, not through challenging them or trying to appear tough. The *quality* of their answers – tone of voice, body language, and facial expression – is as important, or more so, than the specific answer they give. Don't ask these questions in a cadence or checklist fashion: Take some time between each one and ask more questions to be sure that you get enough details. Some suggested questions include the following:

- Has anyone made you angry enough to hit them in the last six months? How about the last year? Have you ever been arrested for assault or for fighting with someone? Notice the nuanced levels of the questions. You are able, here, to assess the patient's familiarity with the legal system, or their lack of truthfulness. By asking "six months," you may get a more manipulative person, who otherwise might lie, to say, "Not in six months," because they think that's all you care about. Or, they deny being convicted for assault, but endorse fighting, which indicates that they went through an entire trial without either paying attention to the charges or becoming interested in the proceedings.
- Tell me what happened. Why do you think this situation occurred? Was there anything you could have done to avoid such a confrontation? The context in which the person was assaultive, what it meant to them, why they thought they had no other options, or why they chose violence first, not last, are all vital information.
- What do you do when someone really makes you angry? What kind of thing might someone say that would make you mad? Among other things, this gives you advanced warning of what the patient's triggers are. A patient might say, "I hate it when I ask to be left alone, and then staff keep at me, telling me I need to talk things out, right now! I hate that!" Predatory intimidators sometimes seize this opportunity to say something vaguely menacing:, "Oh, you don't want to know."
- If you got mad at someone here, what would you do? How would you handle it?
- Is there any situation where you might get so mad that you might want to hit someone, be they staff or patient?
- If you did get mad, how could staff (or "I," in certain cases) help you calm down?

Asking an individual about any history of violence or aggression should not be executed in a checklist fashion, in which a certain number of positives earns a rating of low/medium/high risk. Rather, each criterion is a "gateway" to further questions.

NOTE: This is obviously not a complete list of questions you might ask. These are just a few examples to help you understand the scope and nature of the open-ended questions you need to ask. By asking open-ended questions that require more than a simple yes or no answer, staff can gather quite a bit of critical information. These types of questions can also be used to get the person thinking about their patterns of behavior and their triggers.

CHAPTER 37

What Does Escalation
Look Like?

As a person escalates in their aggressive behavior(s), they are priming their bodies to posture, to intimidate, to fight, or to flee. They can display a variety of behaviors.

Changes of Affect (Their Mood as Reflected in Behavior)

Atypical physical and emotional withdrawal. This is typified by avoiding eye contact, no longer speaking to staff or other patients, or responding only with short phrases and monosyllabic answers. Of course, some people are more naturally withdrawn and reserved: this does not mean that they are readying themselves for an aggressive outburst. I am discussing, here, a heretofore friendly or otherwise engaged patient who lapses into sullen hostility or refuses to engage in conversation.

If you notice a patient behaving in this manner, you should approach them and engage them in order to elicit a response. For example, you may ask, "Hey Tim, every time I do my morning rounds, you say hello and ask me how my day is going, but today, you turned your back and just looked at the floor. Something's bothering you today." Note that you do not ask, "What's going on?" Direct questions will merely give the patient an opportunity to ignore you or reply with simple answers such as "Nothing" or "I don't know." By treating their behavior as meaningful, something about which you are concerned, you are more likely to get a truthful response, such as "I just had a really bad argument with my son on the phone, and don't want to talk about it" or "You know what's going on! You know what you did!" Such a response is the quickest way of ascertaining if the patient is a threat to anyone in your hospital.

Nervousness, anxiety, even fear. Such people usually lash out in defense. They are not looking for a fight; they are trying to protect themselves.

Feeling overwhelmed or disorganized. Patients who speak in repetitive loops, mutter incoherently or pace are displaying symptoms of a chaotic mental state, whatever the cause. Patients in this state can be unpredictable, and they may react to your attempts to communicate with sudden, unexpected aggression.

Hostility. The open expression of dislike, hatred, or threat should immediately put you on guard. A plainly hostile demeanor can escalate into violence quite easily.

Seduction. Seduction is not reserved for just sexual expressions or desires. This is when an individual tries to get you to collude with them. (e.g., "C'mon. It was just a slap. You aren't going to report me for just slapping my kid.") Such individuals' aggression is masked. Things will be "fine" between you if you agree to collude with them; if not, they frequently explode.

Mood swings. This means rapid shifts in mood from, for example, boisterous to morose, then depressed and quiet, and then belligerent (Chapter 7). Such individuals present a particular risk due to their unpredictability and their inability to control their own emotions.

Hypersensitivity to correction or disagreement. Hypersensitive people are very reactive to other people around them. Paranoid people, in particular, may complain of being stared at, watched, or controlled, and feel under constant attack (Chapter 10). When there is no apparent enemy, they will find or even create one. The hypersensitive patient can react aggressively to even the most inoffensive and harmless attempts at communication, particularly if they believe there is any chance that they will be censured or a limit will be set on their behavior. Paradoxically, they do not feel right with themselves unless they discover who is attacking them. In their world, someone always is.

Authority issues. Such a patient becomes very frustrated or outraged, refusing to comply with rules. Limitations on their behavior are, in their view, oppressive or humiliating. Their motto of life can be summed up in the phrase, "No one can tell me what to do."

Electric tension. This is the feeling before a thunderstorm hits. <u>**You must ALWAYS trust this feeling, this intuitive sense that you are approaching a dangerous situation**</u> (Chapter 26).

Cognitive Changes

Cognitive distortions. Cognitive distortions are thinking patterns where the individual makes global, negative assumptions. For example, a patient misses a single meeting at his substance abuse treatment facility and assumes he will be dropped from the program. Therefore, when he sees his case manager, he is already flamed up at the injustice he believes will be perpetrated upon him.

Interpersonal cognitive distortions. This occurs when the person hears the worst possible interpretation in what *another* person is saying. For example: "Tia, you have to start following rules at the hospital, or we may have to ask to you seek services elsewhere." And her response is, "YOU ARE THROWING ME OUT!"

Becoming less and less amenable to conciliation or negotiation. The individual focuses increasingly on dominating the conversation or situation, winning the argument, or taking out their frustrations on the object of their anger rather than trying to find a peaceful resolution. They focus on being "right" and not on the facts. By refusing to consider other perspectives, they value only their own ideas and desires.

Deterioration of concentration and memory. It becomes harder for them to communicate, to solve problems, or to recall past problem-solving skills.

As their information-processing skills deteriorate, **their judgment consequently becomes worse and worse**: They cannot evaluate what is really in their own self-interest.

> ### Example: Impaired judgment
> Frustrated with having to wait for dessert and already in trouble with staff at his group home for several infractions, William overturns the table. That this will result in his being expelled from the group home is irrelevant to him. Depending on his character, all he cares about in the moment is either the ecstasy of violence or the discharge of intolerable tension.

Changes in Patterns of Verbal Interaction

Silence. Potentially aggressive patients may lapse into a morose, sullen silence, often accompanied by hunched shoulders, knitted brows, and glaring at the floor or at other people.

Sarcasm. Sarcasm can be considered hostility shaded with humor or passive-aggressive phrases. The sarcastic person jeers at you, or sneers scornfully, demeaning your strong attributes and highlighting what they perceive as your weak points. Their goal is to make you unsure of yourself or to hold you up to contempt in the eyes of others.

Cold rejection. Your peacemaking gestures are pushed away. The person makes it as clear as possible that there is nothing you can do to change their attitude toward you.

Deliberate provocation. The person says and does things to upset or irritate you. Provocation is a challenge, either to place you in the victim's role (if you do not respond), or to set you up as the "aggressor," through provoking a response on your part that will justify them becoming increasingly hostile, if not violent.

Word games. Such individuals will deliberately twist or misinterpret what you say, trying to confuse you or make you question your own memories of previous encounters. They may act as if it is your fault and that you are provoking them. Everything you say is used as an excuse to further attack you. In making you feel increasingly unsettled, they are grooming you for aggression, for which you, preoccupied with their word games, will not be prepared to respond.

Becoming increasingly illogical. Rather than purposeful, this is a manifestation of increasing agitation. The angry person misunderstands or misinterprets what you are doing or saying. They often go off on a tangent whenever you try to offer calming words or a way to restore peace. Others only focus on one aspect of what you are saying. They become unable to explain what they are doing or trying to say.

Vocal tone. Many angry individuals become increasingly loud and demanding, either with a belligerent tone, as if trying to pick a fight, or simply louder, as if they believe you cannot otherwise hear them.

The latter is caused by their belief that they are not "getting through to you." Others, more calculating, assume a quiet, menacing tone.

Abusive or obscene language. (**NOTE**: spitting, though an action, has the same effect on us and has the same intentions as obscenity.)

- Of greatest concern are verbalizations that are vile and degrading. The aggressor's goal is to make you "less than human," thereby giving them license to be violent. They might not do violence to a human being, but if you are a _____ (fill in the blank), then violence is no more wrong than it would be to exterminate vermin or a wild beast.
- Others use such words as a weapon, to shock or stun, so that you focus on what they say and not on what they are doing (such as moving ever closer, or surreptitiously reaching for a weapon). Imagine someone saying what is, for you, that one unforgivable, absolutely out-of-bounds word. While you are preoccupied with their disgusting language, you don't notice that he is three feet closer to you, and he's surreptitiously picked up the metal ruler that shouldn't have been on your desk in the first place.
- Note, however, that some people, and quite frankly, some of you, use obscenities as adjectives and punctuation. A patient may swear to illustrate their own emotions and ideas, with no intention to use their words as a form of attack. Although your senses may be heightened by their use of vulgarities, you should respond in a calm manner, perhaps asking the patient to refrain from such talk. However, you must be able to distinguish between true aggression and simple speech patterns, as you may end up escalating what was a very benign interview.

Repeated demands or complaints. Of such a person, we often say, "They have an attitude." They may demand that you do things for them, or that you provide an excuse to, for example, their parole officer or doctor, for why they missed an appointment. When you rightly refuse, they may attempt to "turn you in," by telling your supervisor that you are being uncooperative and inattentive to their needs. This person is both trying to leverage others to do things for them as well as looking for a pretext to legitimize what is a pervasive sense of grievance, so that it can coalesce around an issue worth fighting about.

Refusal to comply with rules or directives. In their mind, it is "all or nothing." If they comply, they lose. Only resistance is victory.

Total denial. Such individuals deny either the facts or the implications of what they are doing. They are so angry that reality is irrelevant to them. All that matters is that they are right and you are wrong.

Clipped or pressured speech. Some aggressors attempt to hide their aggression by appearing to be polite – overly so. They often use very formal or stilted language, presenting themselves as being in control when they are actually seething with aggression or a sense of injustice. It is eerie to have such a sense of menace when they are so polite! They are trying to present as someone in control even as they have the pent-up energy of a volcano. This is often the hallmark speech of someone with paranoid traits (Chapter 10).

Implicit threats. As with threatening sarcastic remarks, any implied threats made by a patient must never go unanswered or ignored. This includes people who boast of past acts of violence or who warn you that they might not be able to stop themselves from reacting the same way in the future.

Physical Organization and Disorganization

Facial expressions. These can vary greatly, depending on the person's mode of aggression. Facial expressions will be discussed, as part of a total complex of behaviors, in Section IX. These are among the most significant facial expressions:

- Clenched teeth, usually an attempt to contain or control intense emotions.
- Bared teeth, usually a threat display.
- Frowning can have a variety of causes but is often associated with anger or dissatisfaction with the person the frowner is facing.
- Staring eyes can be an attempt to intimidate, manipulate, or simply target the other as prey.
- Wide-open eyes, looking beyond or through you, can be a manifestation of extreme fear. Psychotic people may be gazing beyond you at visual distortions or hallucinations.
- Biting the lips, usually associated with barely controllable emotions.
- Quivering lips, usually associated with fear or unhappiness.
- Tightening the lips, associated with an attempt to control or contain intense emotion.
- Pulsating veins in the neck, often associated with building anger and rage.
- Dilated pupils, often associated with drug intoxication.
- Avoiding all eye contact, when coupled with other expressions of aggression, is associated with planning an attack, hiding intentions of an attack, or, paradoxically, attempting to disengage so that they will not attack.

Pain in the skeletal muscles and joints. Some people experience pain in the chest, joints, as well as headaches as there is increased blood flow to their tense skeletal muscles. This is sometimes accompanied by a rise in body temperature, resulting in sweating.

Voiding. Some people, when angered, have an urge to void themselves, clearing their bodies for the fight. Nausea and vomiting can occur with reduced blood flow to the gut. Other people feel a need to urinate or an onset of diarrhea. These behaviors notably occur when an individual is in a state of intense fear or otherwise full of adrenalin.

Changes in breathing. Those shifting into hostile, offensive anger often breathe deep in the chest and abdomen. This can be slow or fast, depending on how fast their anger is building. Those going into fearful, defensive aggression usually breathe in a shallow, rapid, and irregular pattern, almost like panting or gasping. Some hyperventilate, breathing so fast and so deeply that they go into a panic state. Such individuals often become violent out of the terror induced by the panic. This panic state is accompanied by a feeling of heart palpitations.

Actions

Tensing or relaxing. Most aggressive individuals become tense and/or agitated. Sometimes people try to discharge the tension by pacing, usually typified by rapid, jerky movements, or even exercising that clearly is not for fun. However, predatory individuals tend to relax when they are preparing for an attack. They are at home with violence, like a tiger or a snake. These individuals sometimes smile while making eye contact with you.

Posturing. Becoming angry, they begin to posture: inflating their chest, pointing a finger, leaning into the other, and/or thrusting their chin forward. This is an intimidation pose rather than a fighting pose. Posturing transitions into ritualized behavior, particularly among men. They go into a stereotypical "war dance," puffing up their chests and spreading their arms to make their torso look bigger, invading their "victim's" personal space, pacing, smacking their fist in their hand, breathing faster, and so on. They may move in quick, jerky starts and stops, making movements toward their victim and then backing off, as if working themselves up to attack.

Positioning. Those looking for a fight or confrontation square off directly in front of their target, while those looking for a victim tend to move to the corner of the person, trying to get an angle on them so that they can attack more easily. This "division" of behavior conforms to the well-known formula of "affective violence" (driven by intent to dominate another) and "predatory violence" (driven by the intention of taking prey).

Fighting pose. A combative stance, unlike posturing, is often a crouch, with the chin tucked in. In other cases, the person brandishes a fist or a weapon. Be aware, however, that those who are most skilled at violence can often attack from a position of complete relaxation.

Trespassing and power testing. An aggressive individual will intrude on your personal space, "accidentally" bumping into you. They may also test your ability to defend yourself or set limits by picking up, mishandling, or even breaking your possessions.

Visually raping. Men, in particular, will use their eyes to trespass on women, running their gaze over their bodies in what can only be considered a "visual rape."

Displacing. Angry individuals may hit, kick, or throw objects in an effort to discharge tension, display threat, or "warm up" to an attack. Another displacement activity is "scapegoating," expressed on living beings rather than on objects. For example, furious that the doctor will not provide him with narcotics, a patient verbally or physically abuses his wife and children.

Making a dramatic scene. The individual "acts crazy," either to get closer to you than you'd let someone who was purposefully targeting you, or to get you so preoccupied with calming them down that you lose sight of larger tactical concerns (like their partner, who is busy stealing medications, or victimizing someone else).

The Edge of Attack

As people continue to escalate, the risk of violence, of course, increases. They shift from anger to rage, becoming harder and harder to reach.

Skin tone. Angry people have a flushed face – the pale skinned turn red, and the dark skinned turn even darker. Blood at the surface of the skin is threat display, as if to say, "See how angry I am!" If people blanch – light-skinned people turn bone-white, and dark-skinned people get a grayish tone – this indicates RAGE; the threat is not potential, it is NOW.

Pacing. Increased pacing, while muttering to oneself, is arousing, bringing oneself closer and closer to the edge or attack.

Calm before the storm. Some people engage in more and more displacement activity, hitting, kicking, spitting, and throwing things. Others internalize all signs of incipient assault. In either case, right before the attack, many people stop breathing for a moment. This is usually accompanied by a "quiet" – the "calm before the storm." The person will "recede" into quiescence or will have a "thousand-yard stare," where they seem to look beyond or through you. It is as if you aren't there. They are very often depersonalizing you and will attack very soon.

The thousand-yard stare

When people go into a "thousand-yard stare," you should, whenever possible, escape. If you are not able to do so, or circumstances demand that you remain, you should strive to bring them "back" to relationship. For example, you can say, "Sammy, listen to me. Put the chair down. You know me. Put the chair down. You don't need that here. You know me, Sam! You *know* me. We can work this out together. Sam, think about what you are doing."

Eerie smile. Some people – particularly, but not exclusively, a person experiencing a psychotic episode – get an eerie smile on their face, one that holds no mirth. This can be driven by a lot of things, but it is sometimes emblematic of the person cutting off human relationship with you and attending only to the voices or impulses within them that urge violence.

Losing it. As the attack is incipient, the person can "lose it," shaking, yelling, and acting berserk.

Explosion and Afterward

The crisis will be some form of assault, possibly explosively violent. Other examples would be stalking or verbal intimidation; however, most often, it will be some kind of dramatic aggression: physical or verbal. As described above, this requires you do whatever you must do to establish safety for yourself and those around you.

After the explosive episode, be it physically violent or not, the aggressor moves to the *resolution* phase in which they gradually, sometimes *very* gradually, return to baseline. Their body relaxes, cognitions improve, and actions are less stereotypical.

After resolution, there is often a *post-crisis depression* that is partly psychological and partly due to physical depletion one experiences after the rush of adrenaline that accompanies any threatening situation. The individual may be remorseful, apologetic, resentful, or merely withdrawn.

As a result of their actions, a number of things might happen next:
- The person might be in the custody of the police, placed in physical restraints, or held in a seclusion room.
- You may have run out of your office, and the person is still inside, enraged: essentially a barricade situation. The police, security, or other staff may have to enter or may have to negotiate with them to surrender.
- The person may calm down, and the crisis is not so severe that he needs to be arrested or restrained. See Chapter 64 concerning the aftermath of aggression.

SECTION VII

De-escalation of
Angry Individuals

CHAPTER 38

Core Principles of Intervention
with Angry People

All of the de-escalation techniques outlined in this section are for angry individuals, between 20 and 95 on the aggression scale. They are not recommended for use with an enraged patient, whom I rate between 95 and 99 on the scale. In fact, using strategies designed for angry people with enraged or violent ones will likely result in a further escalation of the crisis, increasing the risk of injury or assault. Conversely, using strategies and control tactics that are suitable for enraged patients with those who are merely angry can also escalate them *into* rage. In any case, you must first center yourself before stepping into the conflict and establishing control of the situation and the patient. (If you have properly trained in the procedures in Section IV, centering is an almost instantaneous act.) Once the patient is under control and their anger has cooled, you can attempt to resolve the situation that led to the aggression.

Safety is paramount, and it must supersede all other concerns. You may be very aware of the anguish that your patient is suffering. You may find their desire to wreak havoc to be absolutely understandable. Nonetheless, if you do not establish safety for yourself and others, you can be of no assistance to them. This does not mean that you should cease talking, reassuring, or negotiating with them. However, everything you do must have a tactical basis. Even reassurance or validation is in the service of safety. Problem solving must wait until safety is established.

Knowledge is power. You must be aware of anyone with whom your hospital comes into regular contact. This includes patients, family members, and other visitors and even staff. Note any significant changes in both their behavior and their life circumstances. Inform the other people with whom you work, or who may be involved in the patient's care, of the changes you have observed. Check out your perceptions and intuitions with others on your team, and also those at a little distance from the situation. Find out what might be disturbing the individual *before*, not after, a critical incident.

De-escalate, and then solve the problem. Your focus should be on what the patient is doing, rather than solving their problem. You cannot solve a problem with an angry person. Remember, the angry patient sees the conflict as a win-lose proposition. They will view any negotiation or agreement as a loss of power. For this reason, first eliminate the anger and then engage in problem solving.

Presence. Your presence, especially if you are calm and strong, can be enough to calm many people. What sometimes drives the angry person is a sense of being existentially alone. That you are there, perhaps sitting nearby, is sometimes all that is necessary. Proximity is not enough, however. Presence means that you have established through your stance and demeanor an authority that, as quiet as you may be, cannot be ignored.

Watchful waiting. A crisis always requires that you be mindful and aware, so that moment by moment you can decide upon the best course of action. It does not necessarily require that you intervene. Sometimes, all that is necessary is that you remain centered and ready, as the patient calms himself or herself without assistance. This does NOT mean that you ignore them, but in this case the best control tactic is letting the patient control himself or herself. It is like listening to your slightly ill child who begins to fall asleep. You remain aware for any cough or other distress, but you let the child drop off without you.

Trust your hunches. As has been noted throughout this book, you should listen to your intuition and "gut feelings." If you have a vague sense that something is wrong with the patient, or a feeling that he or she might be angry, you are probably right. Once you have such a hunch, you must pay close attention to their behaviors, both verbal and nonverbal. What do you see? How is the patient interacting with other people? Have they been having any recent problems? What is different now from the way they act normally? Remember the characteristic signs and behaviors that this person shows when he or she becomes angry: Are any of those signs showing now?

One point of contact. Only one person, in ideal circumstances, their assigned staff person, should be communicating with the angry patient. This becomes more relevant the angrier they become. Trying to talk to two or more people at once, particularly if *they* are not in complete agreement, will cause the patient to become more and more confused and make him feel surrounded and overwhelmed.

Be what you want them to be. When speaking to an angry patient, you should embody the behavior you desire of them. Speak to them calmly, control your breathing, and maintain an upright and non-threatening posture, all the while remaining ready to respond to any attack. Your hope is that the patient will mirror your behavior and demeanor. This is not an unattainable goal. In crisis situations, people tend to mirror the behavior of the most powerful individual with whom they are interacting. If any staff person is out of control, the patient will feel even more out of control. If you are calm, however, you can take over the situation with that calm.

Courage and respect. <u>These techniques live through your contact with the humanity of the other person, approaching them with courage and with respect.</u> Without this presence, all the techniques in the world will be of no use.

CHAPTER 39

Physical Organization
in the Face of Aggression

How you stand, how you breathe, how you use eye contact, and how you gesture are all essential factors in calming aggressive people. You can say all the "right" things, but if you look like you are afraid, irritated, or unsettled, your verbal interventions will have no effect whatsoever, and the situation will likely get worse. You cannot successfully and safely de-escalate an angry person if you are overwhelmed by your own fear or anger. Such off-center emotions only give the aggressive person power.

Your goal is not a constant state of readiness, going through your day tense and hyper-alert to the slightest threat. Presence, as discussed in the last chapter, is manifest in how you organize your body.

Breathe with your entire torso, not high in the chest. When you breathe rapidly with your chest, you tend to hyperventilate, which "informs" the brain that you're in trouble because you need more oxygen now! Deep, powerful chest breathing, on the other hand, excites the more primal areas of the brain: not flight, but fight. I strongly recommend that you master "circular breathing" as described in Chapter 24. However, for those who aren't able to effectively use circular breathing, or when one has to teach people in a short time, a more simple method[22] is to inhale on a four count, pause your breath on a four count, and exhale on a four count. As described in the last chapter, people tend to calm around people who are powerfully calm themselves. Proper breathing is the quickest avenue toward that end.

Stand or sit? You will most likely be seated in an office setting. Of course, remaining seated when someone is menacing you is very unwise. Other encounters with aggressive individuals may take place in a patient's room, in a hallway, or in a lobby or common area, and you may be standing or sitting, depending on the circumstances. Remain aware of potential avenues of escape, and do whatever you can to keep your exit route open. Do not encumber yourself by holding *unnecessary* items, such as a cup of coffee, paperwork or equipment, while attempting to calm an angry individual.

Stand at an angle to the upset person. This is sometimes called a "blade stance" because you stand with one foot in front of the other, the back foot at a 45-degree angle with some space between your legs. (Don't put two feet in one line as if you are standing on a tightrope!) In this angled stance, your appearance is neither overtly threatening nor fearful. People can actually tolerate your proximity better than if you were standing squarely in front of them, a more confrontational posture. Of course, this stance also allows you to react more easily to an attack.

You can and should also sit with a "blade stance." Sit on the edge of your chair, with your lead foot flat on the floor, your other placed on the ball of the foot. You look interested and attentive, but, in fact, you can easily get up without using your hands or needing to lean forward to get back on your feet.

Are you too close to the patient? (Chapter 26) Medical personnel are almost constantly very close to patients. Even in a psychiatric hospital or group home, staff frequently must help patients with physical tasks and other activities. Do not take this for granted, however. You must never lose sight of the fact that patients, too, have a sense of personal space, and some with a mental illness have an extreme view of this. Some will see any intrusion into their zone as an attack, and they may respond with violence. For everyone's safety, always be tactful when attending to required tasks that involve close proximity or physical contact.

This is all the more important if you are actually trying to calm an angry individual, where your proximity is not for medical or case management tasks, but to control their behavior. As escalation and danger increase, establish the ideal space to create an authoritative presence and to keep out of harm's way, neither too close or too far away. With adults, this is generally two arm lengths' apart. With small children, try to assume a low posture, so that your head heights are equal.

Beyond these basic metrics, don't get so wrapped up in communicating with the aggressive person that you are not aware of their discomfort at your proximity. You will sometimes need far more than two arm lengths. When sensing violation of their space, patients may become more agitated, uncomfortable, or uneasy the closer you get, perhaps shifting back and forth, looking down or away, swaying backward, trembling, or their eyes going flat. Move back so that the patient does not feel pressured or intimidated.

Is the person too close to you? Just as you must be aware if you have moved too close to someone, you also have to warn the angry person when he or she approaches you too closely. Calmly tell the patient that you are happy to talk about their problem, but that they should step back; they are standing too close. You can also say, "I prefer to talk with us farther apart, so I can see you clearly. You are standing too close for me to do that." Many hospital staff are reluctant to do this, afraid, for example, that they will be perceived as uncaring or prejudiced. However, you are showing the other that you are 1) aware of danger, and 2) taking care of yourself. You are also teaching those who, due to their own lack of boundaries, are unconscious of their trespasses.

> **Culture and spacing**
>
> As you know, various cultures have different "rules" about physical proximity and distance. To make matters more complicated, people within any culture are more diverse than you could possibly imagine. Don't assume that someone is close to you "because they are from X culture. Someone *from* X culture may be getting close to you with the intention of harming you. To be sure, you should be aware of cultural conventions. At the same time, such individuals are now living in this culture (wherever you reside) and, therefore, in setting space limits, you are teaching them how to better survive in their new home. Therefore, if someone is too close for your comfort, whatever culture they are from, tell them, tactfully, to move back.

Move slowly and smoothly. Agitated people startle easily. Anything that causes you to move rapidly or in an uncoordinated, jerky fashion, be it overt frustration, anger, fear, or hostility toward the patient, will cause them to become more fearful and/or aggressive, increasing the likelihood of a physical altercation. By breathing and moving smoothly, you hope to induce the person to mirror your actions and attitude.

Use quiet hands. When communicating with an aggressive individual, minimize hand gestures and other movements that could be misinterpreted as an attack. Clasp your <u>wrist</u> with the other hand in front of your body. You can stand this way relaxed for a long time. Don't clasp one hand in the other because you may unconsciously begin wringing them if you get nervous. You will then look scared, and this will frighten people with paranoia, or tempt the predatory to victimize you, in either case evoking the aggression you are trying to avoid. By clasping your wrist, you slightly broaden yourself. You will feel solid rather than nervous. Furthermore, you can easily bring your hands upward to ward off an attack, *without looking like you are ready to do so*. In other words, there is no apparent fight in your stance: just strength. Another benefit is that many of us, when verbally or physically intimidated, don't know what to do with our hands. They tremble involuntarily, or we make unconscious gestures, some of which the other person may interpret either as a threat or as a sign of weakness or fear. Clasping them as described, rather than letting them hang at your sides, keeps your hands occupied.

Use your hands as a calming fence.[23] Fences lend a feeling of security, such as the fence between your property and that of your neighbors. Even while leaning on the fence to talk to a neighbor, we also have a sense of privacy and protection. Similarly, when you extend both of your hands, palms out, in front of you, you establish a boundary between you and your patient. The arms should angle from the body at about thirty degrees, and the hands should be relaxed and slightly curved. If an angry person comes close enough that their body or hands touch yours, there is no doubt that they are intruding within your personal space. Upon making physical contact, most people will back off. People sometimes do not even realize that they are too close until they bump into your "fenced" hands. They step back only when they feel the contact. If they do not step back, this means that they are either no longer aware of personal boundaries, or worse, about to attack.

You can also use these upraised hands to push the person back, "bouncing" yourself backward at the same time, to get some distance from them. *It is important to have the hands and arms relaxed – like a flexible willow branch rather than like iron bars.* The hands should express, in their relaxed calm, that although you are closed off to physical contact, you are open to listening.

You can use your hands as a fence in a more "natural" way by "talking" with them. The hands are held in the same position, but with the backs of the hands forward. You move them in tune with what you are saying – sometimes turning one or both hands forward, or little-finger-edge toward the other person. However, remember to <u>keep your movements slow and small</u>. You are, more or less, rotating your elbows, not swinging your arms from the shoulders. Agitated people will become more so if the person they are talking with is waving their arms in what appears to be threatening or chaotic gestures.

One hand or two?

Paradoxically, holding up *one* hand, although weaker from a combative perspective, is more likely to provoke the patient. Rather than a fence, a single hand becomes the leading point of a triangle, your shoulders being the other two points. Many people experience this as aggression.

Establish eye contact. In most cases, it is best to establish some type of eye contact with the angry individual. As with the other aspects of body language, you must be both unthreatening and unthreatened. Glaring at the patient with hostility or darting your gaze around nervously will just make the patient more ill at ease, and may actually elicit a preemptive attack because they perceive you are about to attack them. To calm someone else, you must show that calm and strength in your own eyes.

There are several exceptions to the eye-contact rule:
- In domestic violence situations, the perpetrator may be assaultive if the victim makes eye contact. The perpetrator hates any manifestation of integrity on their victim's part, and tries to destroy them for having it. <u>Given that this is a totalitarian dictatorship within a home, the only way to improve things is to escape as soon as you can!</u> This is different from the situation of a health or social services professional who is responsible for maintaining both their professional role and the safety of others.
- Some psychotic people find eye contact to be very invasive. Particularly when they are calm, or only slightly agitated, angle your body in such a way that they do not feel confronted or forced to make eye contact with you. Even in these situations, however, you will have to make eye contact to establish control if they escalate into real aggression.
- There is a disinterested "no eye contact" that can be used with *aggressive-manipulative* people (Chapter 59).
- There are some people who are so frightening that you feel apprehensive about making eye contact with them. Others are so chaotic, manipulative, or disorganized that you find yourself

unable to focus on what to do or say when you make eye contact. If this is the case with the person you are dealing with, <u>look between his or her eyes, at the bridge of the nose or the center of the forehead.</u> Remember, the eyes are the only surface area in which living cells touch the air – every other part of the body is shielded by dead cells: hair, skin, nails, etc. When you look in people's eyes, you are revealing who you truly are, and also seeing them in truth. This may be overwhelming for you with some aggressive people. When you look at their forehead, you are literally gazing at layers of dead skin. You will find yourself far calmer, and the other, *if aggressive*, won't be able to tell that you are not making eye contact. You will just appear very strong.

Regardless of the exact nature of the situation, or the other's mental state, do not look away from them altogether. If you turn your attention away from the aggressor for even an instant, you have given them an opportunity to attack. Remember, an attack takes but a split second, especially in close quarters, despite your body positioning and spacing. The aggressor must be aware that *you* are also aware.

CHAPTER 40

The Tone and Quality
of Your Voice

Use a firm, low pitch. In most situations, try to pitch your voice a little lower than is usual for you. You do not need to drop your voice to a baritone or bass, simply a little lower in pitch. It should also be firm and strong. Do not betray any negative or angry emotions; an aggressive person will focus on your tone rather than the content of your words. For example, a bored tone with either impatience or condescension is guaranteed to evoke more anger, not less. If you sound angry, the aggressive person will ramp up their aggression even further, intending to overwhelm you.

When we are upset or frightened, we usually feel out of control of everything, including our own body. Our voices, under stress or intimidation, tend to go up in pitch. On the other hand, you will feel a small vibration in your chest when you pitch your voice lower. When you feel this vibrato in your chest, you get immediate feedback that you have taken back control of your own body. This gives you a sense of power. In addition, a quiet but strong, low-pitched voice communicates that you are in control of yourself and the situation.

Slow down. You should usually speak a little slower than the person you are de-escalating. You are trying to get them to resonate with your slower energy, and also to keep yourself from being swept up in their aggression. Do not, however, speak with an exaggerated slow-motion quality or in such a way that they think you are trying to hypnotize them.

Do not be overly "sweet" or condescending. *Except when you are dealing with small children in distress, do not try to "nurture" them* with a gentle, supportive voice, attempting to convince them that they want to do what *you* want them to do, or desire them to feel. That overly sweet vocal tone seems to say, "I don't have high expectations of you. You are too weak, and I have to care for you like a child." This can provoke the person to regress to a more child-like state, which can easily deteriorate into hysteria or a tantrum, and a tantrum in an adult is usually manifested as chaotic rage. Others, insulted at what they perceive as condescension, become angrier.

Again, your tone of voice should be strong and pitched low in the chest, conveying this message: "I know this is really hard for you. I can't fix it. But I am willing to see if I can help you fix it yourself."

The use of a dramatic voice, **an exception to the rule**. In this case, you *do* make your voice a little louder, and you use drama and charisma to grab their attention. For example, an upset patient believes other patients are laughing at her, so she storms up to the unit desk and demands to see you. You say, "Claire, I <u>see</u> you are upset! I'd be upset too if I thought those people were laughing at me! Now COME ON over here!" Start moving as if you are absolutely certain she will follow (do not, however, turn your back so that you can no longer see her). "Yes, ma'am! C'mon. I want you to tell me EXACTLY what happened! EVERY word. Let's go over here where no one can bother us!" You show her that not only are you giving her your complete attention, but also the drama means that she is important, the center of the action. By moving her somewhere else to talk, you remove her to an area where there are fewer people whom she might victimize or who might agitate her further.

Give verbal commands. For people who are very disorganized or angry, the use of a low-pitched voice may not be effective, as it will not penetrate through fog of their hysteria of agitation. When necessary, give the aggressor clear, firm, even loud commands to cease and desist. This is different from shouting. Do not yell shrilly or with a pleading tone. Be firm and authoritative, letting them know that you are in command, while at the same time offering them an opportunity to negotiate a safe resolution to the crisis.

Reserve the lion's roar for dangerous situations. There are almost no situations where you should yell. There is one exception, however. When the aggressor is moving toward you to attack, or is otherwise presenting immediate danger to another, roar like a lion to startle and freeze their motion momentarily with commands (such as "STAY BACK" or "STEP AWAY") so you can evade, counter, or escape.

- Open your eyes WIDE!
- "Slam" your stomach BACKWARD to try and connect your navel and your spinal column.
- Tighten your throat. (This will be a little painful to some people, leaving a raw throat for the next day, but it's worth it if it saves you or someone else from harm.)
- **ROAR** a command. An important point to remember here is that when an aggressor, already close to you, is moving toward you with hostile intent, do not command them to "stop" or "freeze." They might comply and yet still be too close. Instead, command them to "step back" or "move back." The command "stop" should be used to arrest an action that will result in harm: for example, yell "stop" if an individual is about to assault another person, throw something, or run out into traffic.

CHAPTER 41

Preemptive De-escalation

In many instances, you can use preemptive intervention to calm a patient who seems to be brooding or obsessed with something. This can be anything ranging from a legitimate grievance to a delusion. You avert the crisis before it happens. This technique may be more useful with someone with whom you are familiar, as you will recognize subtle changes in their demeanor that have, in the past, indicated increasing anger. Several tactics may prove helpful in these circumstances.

Greet them and work your way toward the subject. When the person seems to be brooding or preoccupied about something, a grievance or perhaps a delusion or obsession, do not necessarily attempt to address their irritation immediately. Greet them when you approach them: It's common courtesy and shows that you are not avoiding them. In many circumstances, try to draw the patient into a conversation about a benign subject such as the weather, something aesthetically beautiful like the hummingbird that has been visiting the garden in the atrium, the local sports team, or another area of interest to the patient. Such seemingly harmless topics are also an assessment tool. If the patient resists you as you try to refocus them onto something that otherwise would be of interest to them, this informs you right away that the situation is becoming serious, and your primary goal now shifts to attempting to prevent further escalation of their anger and frustration.

Use a "door opener." Begin by stating impartially that you believe something is upsetting them, and that they do not appear to be themselves today. Do not pose your concern as a question, such as "What's wrong with you today?" or "Why do you seem so upset? Is there some sort of a problem?" By asking a question, you give the person an opportunity to simply "close the door" and deny that there is a problem. Instead, use phrases like, "You are really down today," or "Something is going on," or "You looked really sad when your father dropped you off today." These phrases give the person an opening to present their problem to you without seeming to be interrogated. By making an open-ended statement as if it is self-evident, you are implicitly saying, "We are already past the argument whether my perception is real or not. At this point, we are discussing what this perception means to you and to me." Follow this question with *silence*, accompanied by an open inquiring expression on your face, leaving the person space to respond.

Express faith in their ability to solve the problem. If the patient opens up to you and begins discussing the issue, use open-ended questions that require them to respond: "I see why you are so upset, but how do you think you can take care of it?" or "What do you think can be done to fix things with your sister?" Open-ended questions are intended to bring the patient into the conversation by making them consider their options and offer their own solutions. This also gives you openings to suggest other potential solutions their problem or to discuss the possible ramifications of their suggestions.

Questions are only for those who are mildly upset

Questions should only be addressed to a person who is mildly upset or agitated, not to one who is truly angry or enraged.

- Questions are used to "slow down" the person to make them think, but a very angry or enraged aggressor is beyond hearing and processing your questions, let alone being ready to think about alternative solutions.
- If you notice that your questions are making the person angrier, stop asking them, because questions demand answers, and an angry or enraged person will view your continued questioning as a failure to understand their problem or as an abusive interrogation.

Assure them that you want to help. As elementary a suggestion as this might sound, the following illustrates the power of this intervention. A couple begins to argue in the lobby. A nurse approaches and says, "Things can be so stressful here. I don't know what you are going through, but a lot of people have a rough time at the hospital. How can I help you two?" Even if the couple's argument has to do with things they "brought" from home, this intervention is calming. People in the middle of an argument feel like they are in a zone of invisibility – when someone approaches, they realize that they are making a public display. Furthermore, the nurse offers assistance without criticism or without directly focusing on the subject of the argument. She, therefore, ensures that she is not seen as a "part" of the fight.

If the person is only mildly upset, you can, of course, ask questions. Ask what they want or need. If you have a solution to the problem, explain it clearly to them, give them an idea how long it will take and what they should do in the interim.

CHAPTER 42

Across the Spectrum of Anger:
20 to 95 Percent

De-escalation of anger is about resolving everyone's problems. Your problem is the agitated patient, their problem is attempting to obtain a goal. After all, *people become angry and violent because they want something*. Successful negotiations will work to solve everyone's problems, although the angry person is not likely to achieve exactly what they want at the moment.

Mentally ill patients can present a somewhat different de-escalation problem because their fears, concerns, and outbursts may be due to their mental illness, and not necessarily their desire for *something*. In other words, their problems are internal, although this may be difficult to distinguish at the moment of crisis.

This chapter will offer strategies for de-escalating angry individuals. Some are general principles for all de-escalation attempts; others are strategies for specific circumstances. You may only need to use one tactic, but it is more likely that you will use a combination of many. Those skillful at crisis intervention have an ability to shift from one tactic to another, all the while maintaining basic core principles.

General Principles

Honesty is the heart of negotiation. You must be honest and forthright, never making promises (or offering consequences) that you cannot keep, and always keeping the ones you do make. Do not try to fool the patient or agree to their demands in the heat of the moment. If you suggest a solution to the problem, be clear about the limitations. If they do not clearly understand their options, they will later experience a sense of betrayal when they are refused something they want.

If you think of de-escalation as negotiation, then you have the opportunity to achieve a compromise solution to the problem. Since the angry individual is often unlikely to realize their original goal, you can offer them a secondary goal or solution. However, since many people take negotiation as concession, believing they will end up getting everything they demand, you must be absolutely clear with them: "You want X, but X simply cannot happen, so how about Y?" Keep in mind that with de-escalation at this stage of aggression, you are not trying to force the angry person into compliance or capitulation: you are having them *choose* a second or third option because they eventually realize that they are not going to accomplish their original intentions through aggression.

Don't try to win; try to establish peace. Just as you should be honest and forthright when de-escalating an angry person, so too should you be respectful following the successful resolution of the event. Regardless of their motivations, you should strive to help the individual save face. Try to resolve the situation so that they can separate with their pride intact, increasing the likelihood that, even if they have not achieved their original goal, they will at least have a certain amount of respect for the professional way that you handled the situation. If they feel cheated or betrayed, they will likely be noncompliant in the future due to the personal animosity they feel toward you as an individual, and the hospital as an institution.

Be aware that word of your behavior travels quickly both inside the hospital and outside in the larger community. Never forget that your patients and their families talk to each other – all the time. If you treat someone in a disrespectful manner, or go back on your word, your reputation will precede you when dealing with others, leading to confrontational relationships before you ever meet. The contrary is also true.

There <u>are</u> times you must win

The phrase "Don't try to win, try to establish peace" is in reference to the de-escalation of anger, NOT to the terrible situation of a life-and-death struggle. In the latter, your intention must be "I will win. I will go home to my family."

Make haste slowly. As described in Section IV, *your* attitude is an essential component to de-escalation. The individual in crisis believes there is no time left. If you also believe there is no time, you are now enmeshed within the same crisis, and you will not be able to act as a stable person to help the patient back to a peaceful state. Consider the deliberate actions of an emergency room doctor or paramedic out in the field. They are calm and act with no wasted motion. **Above all else, try to move into the situation with the attitude that you have all the time you need.**

You should maintain a powerful calm, not only in your attitude but also in your actions. The patient may interpret any sudden move on your part as an attack. Therefore, you attempt to "template" the angry person to your calm: by breathing smoothly, by speaking clearly and with a low voice, and by moving in a smooth coordinated way, you are trying to draw the angry individual "into your orbit."

Be professional. This phrase can sound like an empty cliché: poorly thought out and poorly defined. "Professional" means that you clearly maintain some emotional distance from the patient and their family, and that your interactions are circumscribed by your professional responsibilities. Some inpatient personnel act too much like a friend to the patient. Professional distance gives the patient a clear understanding of the true nature of your relationship with them. For example, limit setting, acceptable from a professional, can be experienced as something a friend has no right to do.

Stay concise and clear. Use easily understandable words, and keep it simple, using only one thought in a sentence, rather than long run-on, multi-leveled paragraphs.

Create an exit plan for both of you. Part of any problem-solving strategy is how you will disengage, and what each of you will do once you've done so. The angry person should have a clear idea of what he or she needs to do, how the problem is expected to end, what will result from the solution, and what they should now expect from you.

Create a private space. Create a private space without an audience, if at all possible. If people are already present, try to separate the agitated person from the onlookers.
- Terrified people may be frightened by the onlookers.
- Enraged people or predators might become excited by the crowd or begin to attack other people.
- Bluffers may be afraid they will lose face. Therefore, in front of others they will "have to" aggress.
- Manipulators will use the crowd to their own advantage.

Do not reward aggression

Don't turn the "private space" into a reward. Try not to usher the aggressive person into an office, particularly of someone of "higher rank." That gives the aggressor status and implies that his aggression got him the reward. Move to a neutral space whenever you can. This can be a common room or even a space outside the building.

Try to get the person to sit rather than stand – Pacing and stomping around is stimulating. You are also more ready to fight when you are standing. In addition, we associate sitting and talking, and even more so, sitting and listening, with peaceful communication. When we sit together, we find ourselves more ready to solve problems and figure things out, not act things out.

Strategies for Specific Circumstances

Don't rush in when the situation is unclear or ambiguous. When you approach a situation that appears potentially volatile or problematic, do not simply rush in and try to take over. Center yourself first (Section IV). Get other staff together, if you can, to quickly discuss the best thing to do. Remember, your patient may be trying to calm down, and if you simply run in and try to take over, you may interfere with their attempts to control and soothe themselves. In other circumstances, they may perceive themselves to be under attack, because when they are preoccupied with their internal de-escalation process, your sudden intervention will surprise them.

This principle is particularly important in crowded situations. Here, there is an even greater reason to advance with measured steps; you must understand what is going on and who the "players" are on the scene. The person you perceive as the angry individual may be, for example, a victim of someone else's taunting or assault, and as you focus on him or her, you can be blindsided by the real aggressor.

Don't touch the irritated person hoping to calm them down. Outside of physical restraint procedures, which can be necessary when a patient is either on the edge or already violent, there are very few situations where touching an angry person will make the situation better. Such situations do exist, particularly with distraught children, but in most situations do not put your hands on angry people, even if you intend to comfort or mollify them.

Demonstrate empathy. Empathy is not the same as sympathy, that feeling of sorrow for another person's plight. Empathy simply means that you grasp, approximately, what the other person is experiencing, based on their physical organization, what they say, and how they say it. You can express empathy through phrases like, "I understand you are . . . " or "What you are saying really makes sense," or "I imagine I'd feel the same way . . ."

> **Over-empathy will result in the patient becoming more rather than less angry**
> Do not overuse empathic phrases or you will sound like a parody of the worst kind of counselor. The angry person will become extremely irritated with you; the more antisocial or predatory person will perceive you as weak.

Help them get it off their chest. Sometimes people simply have to say their piece. There is no need to problem solve: all you need to do is listen with a powerful, quiet attention. Given an opportunity to speak, they will. The only real requirement here is that you do not begin to intervene or offer suggestions until the person has been able to say his or her piece.

It is often necessary to encourage the person to speak in more detail, particularly if they are so upset that you can't understand what they are talking about. Some people rush through their explanation, expecting to be cut off. (That expectation, of course, fuels even more anger.) Some are so caught up in the situation that they assume you understand, and, therefore, only give sketchy details. Other people are so agitated that they don't make much sense. Say to them, "Tell me more about that," or "Take your time. I really want to know what is going on. There's no hurry."

> **You must differentiate between a person "getting something of their chest" and venting**
> Venting can be viewed as a form of verbal aggression, albeit toward another individual or entity who is likely not present. The danger with allowing an angry person to vent for any length of time is that venting, in and of itself, becomes arousing to the person. As they begin talking about the issue at hand, they can become more agitated, and, hence, aggressive. Venting must be de-escalated and controlled like any other type of anger or rage (see Chapter 45).

Filter out the static and leap ahead to the objective. Some patients present a particular problem – over-inclusiveness. These individuals do not merely tell you what is wrong. They will, in addition, tell you their life story, perhaps, or voice obsessions and delusions that either do not pertain to the current problem or obscure just what the problem is. It is often necessary to cut such people off – and focus specifically on the current problem.

> ### Examples: Filtering out the static and controlling a cascade of words
> - "Douglas, you are telling me too many things at the same time. I know you need help, but I don't know what kind of help. What is bothering you *right now*?" You will have to be calmly assertive, because the individual's delusions or obsessions are so fascinating to them or so dominant that they easily lapse back into them. "Douglas, stop. You may not tell me more about the Punic Wars. Not one more word about that. I know you are also upset with Francine. You and I need to speak about that now."
> - You may have to define your scope of work. "Jesse, I do not know anything about alternative energy or about geology. I am your nurse. We must talk about your medications. Remember, your prescription was changed. I know alternative energy is a very important subject, but you will have to discuss that with other people who know more about that than I do. We have to talk about your medicine."

Interrupt to clarify misunderstandings. If the person voices a misunderstanding of the situation and they are not so agitated that they can accept an interruption, you can sometimes interject and solve the dispute, saying something like, "Just a moment, Madeline. Before we go on, let me tell you something important. You are not being sent home today. The doctors think your recovery has been a little slow and that you *should* stay for at least three more days."

> ### Clarification is not argument
> Clarifying a misunderstanding is not the same as your interjecting to argue that they don't understand your position or attempting to save face by explaining why you did what you did. This strategy is used specifically to correct a patient's misunderstanding that is the primary cause of their anger.

Remind them of what they know (past experiences, coping strategies, and rules). This strategy is specifically for people at lower levels of anger. Particularly when the person is only mildly angry, the best thing to do can be to remind them of what they already know, but have forgotten, due to their anger. Remember, this should not come off as scolding! You are not criticizing them for forgetting something – you are supporting them by reminding them what they do when the best aspect of themselves are active and aware.

- *Remind them that all problems can be worked out by talking.* There is no need to throw things or hit. Remind them that you've done it together in the past and are happy to do it again.
- "Remember the last time you . . ." Remind them of a positive outcome, not a negative one! Help them remember how they succeeded in extricating themselves from such a problem before.
- Remind them of what you or other staff have taught to help them deal with difficult situations – everything from walking away, exercising, writing ideas in a journal – whatever has worked for that person in the past. "Anna, before we continue, remember what we talked about regarding breathing. You learned that problems are much harder to solve when you are breathing fast. I've got plenty of time. Go ahead and do your breathing for a couple of minutes. I will count for you so you can pace your breath. Signal me with your hand, like this, if you want me to count slower. I'll wait. Then, when your breathing is slower, we'll talk."
- Beyond coping strategies, patients should have already been clearly informed of such rules as no violence, no intoxication, and no attempts to solicit romantic relationships, upon entry into your hospital. There are many times when the best thing to do is to simply remind the person what they either have forgotten, or would like to ignore. If not reminded, or, in the latter case, given license, they will continue to break the rules.

Team up with them, creating an alliance. When you team up with the angry person, you make the situation a common problem. This is most effective when the person sees you as, at least, a potential ally. It does not work well in a situation where the angry person views you as an adversary. Teaming up requires not only words, but also action. Your offer should include a request that the person does something with you; if they refuse, it is unlikely that you will be successful with this tactic.

Examples: Creating an alliance
- "Let's you and I sit over here." "Yes, we do have a problem. Let's see what we can do to figure this out."
- Ask people to come with you down the hallway to continue the discussion because people in the lobby might misinterpret the loud voices and get frightened, overhear private information, or choose to involve themselves. One way to do this is to make a request: "Shall we go outside the building where I can talk with you without anyone bothering us?"

One aspect of teaming up is finding something – anything – that the two of you can agree upon.

Examples: Finding something to agree upon

- "Look, I know things have been hard, but your kids are here. Let's move over here so they don't have to hear this."
- "Yep, I have no doubt whatsoever that you are angry. Furious. Let's get a drink – coffee? Tea? Soda? And you tell me about it."
- "I am aware you don't agree with me, and I don't think we are going to get anywhere further now. How about we speak tomorrow, and you tell me after thinking about it, if you still disagree." (Note here that the agreement is to separate and return, not agree with your position.)

Simpler examples:

- "Will you, at least, think about it?"
- "Does that make sense to you?"
- "I understand you disagree here, but do you see how I might come to that sort of idea?"

Suggest a separation. Suggest that the two of you take a break and promise to return to the subject later. Phrase it in a way that puts the responsibility on you: "I'm having trouble concentrating. Let's both of us take a break, and we'll talk about this later. If we continue, I'm not going to make much sense, and nothing will be resolved. Let's set a time. It's two o'clock now. Let's talk again at four."

Do not tell the person to take a "time-out," because angry people may believe you are patronizing them and talking to them as if they were children. Disengaging is particularly useful when you both are at an impasse, and continued discussion will simply increase the level of frustration between you. It is also the right thing to do when you feel flooded: helpless to get through to them, overwhelmed by emotion (any emotion), or confused.

Caution! Separation doesn't mean it's over

Many people who choose separation feel a sense of relief that the confrontation is over and, because they feel better, assume that the problem is solved. Understand that the person you separated from may be fuming, planning his or her responses when you reinitiate the discussion. Their anxiety and anger may begin to increase the longer they wait. When you do not reengage, either at a promised time, or worse, if it was left "open" when you two would talk about things again, the other person interprets this as a sadistic control tactic on your part, making them wait, even "making me come to you to ask for a little attention!" To make matters even worse, the people whose default is "out of sight, out of mind" often act surprised when the other reinitiates the conversation or confrontation.

If you initiate the separation, give the other person a clear idea of when you will reinitiate it, and keep your promise.

Take responsibility. Sometimes the best thing to do is to take over: sum up the situation, tell the client or other person to do something, such as wait in the lobby, go back to their book or the TV, and promise that you will take care of the situation. This requires you to state the following:

- A realistic idea of what to expect.
- A specific time when you will return with results.
- A promise that if you are not able to accomplish what you have committed to within that time, either you or your delegate will return to the person with a progress report.
- If you do not follow these steps, the individual will, very likely, become anxious and then angry when things seem to be taking too long or if a long-awaited solution doesn't conform to their fantasies, which have time to percolate in the interim.

Give praise for their good ideas. Don't be over-effusive, but highlight any positive moves the person makes. If they find this rewarding, this will encourage them to offer more productive solutions. It is important not to merely praise them, as if a few compliments will solve everything. "Ride" the praise into a problem-solving solution.

Example: Praising an idea

"I like that idea. I think we can make it work. What we have to find out first, however, is if we can get permission for you to use that room. You are absolutely right. You are in a much better mood when you can play your guitar. You need to understand, however, that I do not make decisions on room allocation. So let's you and I think of an alternative, if that room is not available."

If they try to disengage, let them. Assaults commonly occur when one person tries to disengage, often doing so with yelling and obscenity in the process, and the other person insists on working things out *right now*. This is almost always a mistake. That person is leaving to calm down. The only time you might insist you stay engaged is when you have a legitimate concern that the person's leaving might result in harm to them or to someone else.

About self-revelation. It is occasionally helpful to describe a situation you went through when you experienced something similar: fear, embarrassment, anger, etc. You must be careful and use this strategy very sparingly, as there are a number of ways it can backfire:

- The angry person should not feel that you expect to be comforted. You are demonstrating your understanding, not expressing a demand that they take care of you the same way you take care of them. If they perceive any pressure to take care of you or feel sorry for you, you will probably be vehemently and angrily rejected.
- Self-disclosure can also trigger anger in some individuals because they feel that you, in telling your story, are pushing them off their "stage." The patient essentially says, in outrage, "This is for me! You are taking the only thing that is just for me."

- You can implicitly trivialize the other's distress. When you say you went through something similar, you can, if not careful, also imply, "And here you are, all messed up while I, with the same problem, am doing fine."
- Finally, if you make a spurious comparison, the person will either blow up or blow you off. To use a silly example, if someone tells you about the death of their child, you should not try to establish common ground by revealing your pain at the death of your cat.

Ask what they think would make things better. Ask for their ideas on what would make things better then repeat it aloud "just so I've got it clear." This can help someone feel like you are taking things seriously.

- Surprisingly often, the angry person has a wonderful idea for a solution. But you sometimes get so involved in solving the problem for them that you neglect to ask.
- People sometimes get stuck on irrational ideas that they won't let go of until they propose it to another person. The utter absurdity of an idea can only be grasped when they hear it coming out of the their own mouth or they see the look of astonishment on your face after they say it. At the same time, make sure that you convey that you are truly listening and trying to understand, not mocking them.

Try to acknowledge some or all of the other's point of view. You do not lose any power when you concede someone is right, when, in fact, they are. However, an angry person, particularly one who uses manipulation as a strategy, can interpret this as submission and escalate further, so your concession should be made assertively and strongly.

Example: Set parameters – only acknowledge what is true or right

"Roger, you are right here. No, listen to me carefully. I agree with your complaint about the noise, but I do not agree with what you are planning to do about it. Yes, you *are* right, and therefore, I want to help you. But I will not help you lose your room here, which is what is going to happen if you continue to yell and throw things."

Distract. Particularly with young or cognitively impaired people, it is often best to simply distract them. This is sometimes useful even with people who are experiencing a delirium state, where you distract them long enough so that they can be safely restrained. The anger of disorganized people is often driven by inchoate feelings and sensations, rather than by what they are thinking. If you can change the focus of their attention, their anger can dissipate. This can include food or drink, or sometimes simply pointing something out that is fascinating. "Look at that hummingbird! I haven't seen one all year. What a beautiful green and blue color!"

Giving something has a number of ramifications beyond distraction. Let us consider offering food, juice, or a toy, or in some milieu where smoking is still allowed, a cigarette.[24] When you give someone a gift that is meaningful to them, this transaction has symbolic importance far beyond the distraction, the monetary value, or the momentary pleasure. For most of humanity, a gift accepted is an emblem of a relationship that should not be violated.

Humor. The ability to see a situation from another perspective can sometimes work like magic with angry people. <u>However, you must be very careful: it only is helpful when the person is at low levels of escalation rather than strong anger</u>. If they are too upset or agitated, their response to a joke or humorous comment is likely to be, "You are making fun of me," or "This is serious. You think this is a joke?"

Example: A strategic joke

Many years ago, when I was a member of a mixed-race group, one of the men, provocative, and with a history of assaults, started singing a little song: "I got a bullet here for every white man here, because every one should die." I smiled at him and said, "That won't work on me. I can only be killed by a silver bullet, followed by garlic and a stake through the heart." I looked at him blandly, and he gave me a momentary hard stare. Then we both broke into laughter and the atmosphere in the room lightened considerably.

Apologize. When you hurt the other person's feelings, have to break a promise, or otherwise do something wrong, APOLOGIZE! It will not compromise your authority. It shows that you are a gracious and strong enough person to take responsibility for your own mistakes:

- If the person has a good reason to be upset or a legitimate complaint, accept the criticism and apologize.
- If the person is partially right, concede that point, but continue to differentiate where you are responsible and where you are not.
- If someone will not accept the apology or concession, or is making unreasonable demands, do not continue with more and more apologies. If the first apology is rejected, reiterate in a stronger voice: "I meant what I said. I am sorry for what I did." But if the person continues to berate you, then say, "I have already apologized and I meant it, so I can't do it again. *(pause)* James, we have fifteen minutes left in our meeting. We can use that time to work on other things or we can end it now. But as I have already apologized, there is no point in doing so again. It will not help to just repeat myself."
- If you cannot disengage, use other tactics – depending on their level and mode of aggression.

Use tactful speech. It is easy to become overly familiar or patronizing with people. Your speech, though on the same wavelength, should always be a *little* more formal than the other person's speech. Genuinely courteous behavior can often circumvent the aggression cycle from occurring at all. On occasion, you can be almost ceremonial: "Sir, how about if you come up here, sit down, and we'll talk?"

It is sometimes very powerful to use their family name – Mr., Ms., etc. This formality can, in many cases, change the tenor of a situation. Just as one automatically lowers one's voice when entering a courthouse, many people similarly change their behavior when addressed in a more formal manner.

Give two choices, both of which, in fact, are positive as far as you are concerned. Here are some examples: "Do you want to give the book to me or put it down over there?" or "Do you wish to continue to talk about this now, in a low voice, or would you like to discuss it peacefully tomorrow?" This gives the individual a sense of control, although, in fact, either one of the alternatives is acceptable to you.

Withdraw strategically. There are some times when you absolutely CANNOT engage with the person. For example, let us imagine that your patient wants to initiate an argument while some of the other residents are present. Your treatment facility has been "hot" for days, and any conflict draws residents who often do their best to provoke the action.

- **State firmly**, "I'm not going to discuss this right now." Do NOT say, "I don't want to discuss this."
- **Immediately give the reason**: "I *will* talk about this, but not right now. This isn't the time or the place. Something as important as this shouldn't be news for the rest of the unit. I respect you too much to have the other residents listening to your private business."
- **Set conditions when you can discuss the problem**: "We can go out on the porch in half an hour. We can sit down and talk about it until we figure things out."
- **Disengage, do not talk about it further**. Do not make eye contact that would indicate that you want to discuss it further. However, keep aware with your peripheral vision and your ears wide open in case the person becomes aggressive or even violent.

Beyond the above form of disengagement, there are times, such as when confronted by an individual who is much more powerful (who may be armed or on display in front of his confederates), where a "tactical" retreat is the very best means of control. You take the target of his rage, *you*, out of the picture. You can gather your thoughts and return later, when you feel in control. You can also gather reinforcements or call for help.

CHAPTER 43

Diamonds in the Rough:
Essential Strategies for
De-escalating Anger

Codes for Living: Following the Access Route

People live by codes. Some of those codes are based on the culture into which they are born, and others are based on the culture or lifestyle they adopt. Some of these codes are passed down within a family. Other people may choose in reaction or resistance to the codes they were bequeathed, while some develop their own credo, unique to themselves. Mentally ill individuals may develop an eccentric set of rules congruent only with their mental illness or character disorder.

The heart of their code can be a phrase of one or two words, a core metaphor that sums up their deepest values. The phrase is often interwoven throughout their speech. This is especially true with an angry person whose reason(s) for outrage is their belief that their code is being threatened or compromised:

- They perceive that others are demanding they violate their code.
- They believe they are facing a choice that forces *them* to violate their code.
- They take offense when others do not conform to their code.
- Another's actions require them to respond, lest they violate of their code.

Angry people will often proclaim their values and code for living in their explanation or tirade. You should be able to identify their core metaphor in one or two words or phrases.

Examples: One's code reflected in one's speech
- "I'm a man. He can't talk about me that way."
- "Think of how I feel. If someone did that to you, wouldn't you be upset?"
- "Are you saying I'm not going to get paid? Whether you like or not isn't the issue; you made a promise to pay me when it was done!"
- "I was standing there. Everyone was looking at me, talking about me. I was just 'out there,' and I couldn't make it stop."

Take some time to think about the core metaphor of these individuals. You should be able to delineate the access route in one or two words. What is most important to each of these people in the above examples? Notice that in the last two examples, a code has "coalesced" into a specific issue – in the third example, into debt and promises, in the fourth, humiliation.

Using the code to reach the person – The code is an access route to the person. When you incorporate it in your response, you are recognizing their values (however, misguided or antisocial), and the other person feels understood. That is what most angry people, particularly those who are urban street oriented, mean by "respect." This connection, however tenuous, allows you to work with the angry person toward a resolution. Another way to think of this is that you are filtering out the static and noise to get to the real music. Consider these examples:

- If you discern that personal integrity is a core issue of concern to a man, frame your responses and suggestions with the same theme: "I wouldn't want people talking about you as a man who can't control himself."

- To a young man who believes someone treated him with "disrespect," you could say, "I can see how angry you are. I'd be angry too if someone said that to me, but if you try to hurt him, you'll end up losing. You'd lose your room and you'd be out on the street. Yeah, I know you think he *disrespected* you, but if you assault him, you would be letting him '*own*' you. He says three words, and your response means you lose your room here? No, I'm not saying to let it go. Let's see what we can do, so you win in a real way, so you keep your room and your self-respect."

- Sometimes a core metaphor is situational, something as ostensibly benign as the weather: "Look, Frank, it's a hot day, I'm tired, and I guess you are too. I don't care who's right here, really. I just want to finish this paperwork so you can get that appointment with your psychiatrist. The computers are down, so we have to figure out some other way to get you an appointment. Gosh, these hot days are awful. Here we are, all stressed out just cause we're both hot and tired."

- A mentally ill person, in particular, can get so focused on an issue that they get "tunnel vision," and it is all they can think about. In effect, the problem defines their existence at the moment. "You are absolutely right, those meds are disgusting. They must taste terrible, but if they didn't work so well, I'd never tell you to take such foul-tasting things. But they do work, don't they?" (Of course, knowing this may help you design effective treatment plan interventions, such as offering applesauce or some other beverage to counteract the bad taste of the medications. But the patient will probably not be interested in such a solution unless they clearly believe that you understand how awful the meds taste.)

- Here, the person's outrage is based on his code that he is a helpful person: "Of course you are upset! You were trying to help Esther, and you made a simple suggestion. She told you to shut up. She didn't see that you were simply trying to help. She didn't understand that you weren't bossing her around. You were just trying to be helpful!"

Charting the access route

If you understand the personal codes by which your patients' live, you'll have a roadmap for lining yourself up with what matters most to them. For those who maintain chart notes concerning your patients, I recommend that you have a special place in your chart, easily accessible, where you write down the patient's code for living. This is often placed in the case plan, in the section on effective interventions. Be sure to highlight the access route in some way so that the reader of the chart clearly understands how important it is to the patient.

Break the Pattern

We often find ourselves in the same arguments over and over again, and often with different people! In order to detect any patterns or behaviors that may have negatively affected your communication with patients or other people, you can easily perform a review of you own actions and responses in past disputes, noting, in particular, your "hot buttons" (Chapter 23). Honest self-reflection will reveal any patterns of behavior, personal style, even *your* personal codes that may have had a detrimental effect on your relationship with a particular individual or group of similar people. As with those in any occupation, you can get "caught in a rut" that only deepens with prolonged interaction with aggressive people, especially those who are mentally ill.

There are many occasions when an aggressive person, set on conflict, attempts to enmesh you in an inescapable system. Consider the following:

- Aggressive man: "What are you looking at?" "Nothing," replies the intimidated person. "What? You called me nothing?"
- Aggressive man: "What are you looking at?" "I just looked in your direction," replies the intimidated person. "What! There's something on my face you don't like? Or are you just calling me ugly?"

Effective de-escalation is a two-way street, contingent upon your ability to remain in control in the face of a potentially dangerous situation. Although you may not be able to change the aggressor, you can change yourself. As a professional, you must not take personally any insults or disparaging remarks made by the angry person. Doing so will only make things worse, with the two of you ramping up, back and forth, in reaction to the other.

Any time you alter the dynamics of the communication system between you and another person, you change everything. For example, if you flinch whenever the person swears, resolve to keep a peaceful body. If you become defensive when the person calls you a name, do not argue or object – change the subject instead. If you typically start lecturing when verbally attacked, keep an open frame of mind this time.

At times, however, you may be forced to more dramatically break the pattern of interaction between you and an aggressor by doing or saying something that makes it impossible to continue the dispute. In many cases, you will use a dramatic voice or display somewhat uncharacteristic or unexpected behaviors. This technique is not recommended for "routine" episodes of de-escalation, and most definitely not for an opening in any encounter. However, jumping out of the system can be effective because many aggressors expect their victims, including hospital personnel, to react in a somewhat predictable manner to their displays of anger and/or violence. By reacting in an unanticipated manner, you can throw the aggressive person off balance. Here are a few examples of breaking the pattern:

Example #1: Breaking the pattern

A police officer was arresting a drunk when he called her a word that, more than any other, makes many women incensed. With a look of puzzlement on her face, she said, "Jimmy, do you spell that with a K or a C?"

"K," he replied.

"Jimmy, if you are going to use big-boy language, you should at least know how to spell it. It starts with a C."

"It does? Damn, they didn't teach me that one in school."

Example #2: Breaking the pattern

A very aggressive, manic individual, after capering around my office while verbalizing very dangerous fantasies, whirled around and said to me, a grin of delight on his face, "You are scared, aren't you?" I blurted out, "Yes, I am." (This, a story from early in my career, was clearly a mistake I wouldn't make today.) He then started to stalk menacingly toward me. Realizing I was in danger, I jumped up and yelled in a dramatic voice, "You know what I'm scared about? I'm scared what's happening to kids today! They are being murdered in wars throughout the world. But we don't even have to go that far! They are cutting school lunches and little children who go to bed hungry are not even being fed in schools! I'm scared what's happening to kids today!" With a look of shock on his face, he dropped into a chair and said, "I like kids. What are we going to do about that?"

Example #3: Breaking the pattern

A police officer was arresting a hostile man, who was trying to avoid having handcuffs put on him. The methamphetamine-intoxicated man yelled an obscene accusation about the officer's assumed sexual predilections. The officer jumped back and said, "Goddamn it! You make one mistake twenty years ago, and they never let you forget!" The man held up a hand and said, "Whoa, whoa brother. That's OK. These things happen to everyone. It's OK," and turned around, offering his hands to be cuffed.

Example #4: Breaking the pattern

A man came into a clinic, drunk and belligerent, looking for a fight. I came out and said, "Man, WHAT have you been DRINKING? Me, I like Ten Canes Rum. Whoa, *<holding up two hands and yelling boisterously>* not your turn yet! I'm talking about my rum! Ten stalks of sugar cane for one bottle of rum. It is SWEET as sin and gold as a tiger's eye. You like whiskey, huh? What kind?" He blearily looked at me and said, "Whiskey." I said, "What KIND of whiskey? I need to know WHAT you have been drinking! Man, I love my rum. I go home, take two ice cubes, and put them in a glass. When the rum hits that ice, I hear a crack as clear as the bell in a church and I know everything is going to be all right!" Within five minutes, we were sitting on two chairs, laughing and talking about our favorite drinks.

Example #5: Breaking the pattern

A case manager was visiting a home with a woman and her very dangerous son, who was suffering from schizophrenia. However, he was never violent in the presence of his mother, so she believed she was safe. The three of them were baking cookies, when his mom suddenly said, "We need more milk," and bustled out of the house to go to the corner store before the case manager could tell her to stop. The young man began glaring at her, saying, "I know who you are. You are a serial killer. You deserve to die because of all the people you killed." He grew increasingly agitated. The case manager, keeping the table between them as he stalked toward her, replied, "You are right! I am a cereal killer! This morning, I drowned my Cheerios in milk, and yesterday I crunched my Grapenuts between my teeth. I kill cereal every morning for breakfast." He tried to return to his menacing theme, but she maintained a cheerful "rant" about the breakfast cereals she ate. Finally, he said, "You don't make any sense at all! You aren't doing this right!" His mother soon returned, the son pretended nothing happened, and the case manager left soon afterward. (In future meetings, she got a guarantee that the mother would not leave the house while she was there.)

Determining the time and necessity for breaking the pattern may seem like magic, but instead, this is a highly intuitive skill that is developed with time and experience. Because future behavior is unpredictable, you cannot prepare an array of specialized catch phrases to disarm an aggressive patient. This technique is pure improvisation, like jazz or rap, grounded in a powerful calm. If you consciously try to be creative, or if you are excited about what a cool or funny thing you are about to say, you may indeed say something witty, but it will be at the wrong time, to the wrong person. When you are centered, in control of yourself, and with the mainline skills of de-escalation at hand, such improvisation will simply emerge.

Silence

Sometimes the most powerful thing you can do is to keep silent. Be sure that you are not being passive-aggressive, fuming in silent anger, or appearing to ignore or dismiss the angry person. Instead, you should powerfully, quietly wait. Such silence can evoke curiosity, anxiety or a desire for a response. Keep your facial expressions calm, your posture centered, and carefully listen. Nod your head calmly as you listen, doing so slowly and intermittently. In many cultures, including the United States, nodding your head too rapidly indicates that you want the other person to hurry up and finish, or worse, just shut up. Silence, however, is not that easy, particularly for the person who is suffering the brunt of another's anger. There are three ways to listen silently, and two of them will escalate people even further.[25]

Contemptuous silence. You are tired of the dispute, or may be tired of the person. You fidget, you sigh, and most significantly, you roll your eyes upward to one side. You twist one corner of your mouth. In almost every culture, this facial expression and behavior express an attitude of contempt and is guaranteed to provoke anger, even rage, in others.

Stonewall silence. When you stonewall, you ignore the other person or otherwise make it clear that you wish they would be quiet. Your demeanor shows that you have no interest in what they have to say or why they are saying it. In social services or health settings, you can inadvertently appear to do this when you are inputting data, simultaneously listening on the phone or to another conversation, or taking notes. Such dismissive behavior, whether intended or not, evokes incredible anxiety, even anguish, in the other person who wants to communicate with you, only to find that there's a "wall" in the way. They will do anything to "get through to you," including trying to tear down that wall.

The right way to listen silently: interested silence. When you have been listening well, angry people often interrupt themselves to ask, "Aren't you going to say something?" or "Don't you have any ideas?" If they continue to talk and talk, *you* may have to interrupt them.

Do this by advancing a hand slightly at your waist level or a little higher, fingers curved, palm down (you don't want the person to interpret your hand movement as a "shut up" gesture). You should also lean toward the patient slightly, indicating that it's your turn to speak.

After interrupting the angry person, the first thing you should do is to sum up your understanding of what he or she just said: this proves that you were, indeed, listening to them, and are interested in solving their problem.

CHAPTER 44

Paraphrasing: the Gold Standard with Angry People

Paraphrasing may be the most important technique for calming angry people. This technique is also sometimes referred to as "active listening" or "mirroring." The term paraphrasing is used here to highlight some important differences between my preferred method and that of many others.

"Mirroring" often entails repeating word-for-word what the other person is saying. This can, at best, be irritating, and can easily be seen as taunting or mocking. The term "active listening" often carries a certain ideological baggage as well. Through active listening, many clinicians try to establish a nurturing relationship with the other person, with the intention of either making them feel better or allowing them to emote freely, under the theory that they have negative emotions/energy pent up and only a "safe, holding environment" will allow them the freedom to express themselves. This is, in a subtle way, manipulative. Talking to another person as if they were fragile may make them feel so, or they may feel that you are *trying* to make them feel weak. In either event, this can elicit "contact regression,"[26] where the person becomes childish, angry, or even enraged.

Paraphrasing, on a more matter-of-fact level, simply establishes that you are truly listening and have understood what they have said. You sum up in a phrase or sentence your understanding of what the patient has just said, as disorganized or confused as that might be. If you paraphrase accurately, you've established that you've "got it" so far, and the patient does not have to repeat himself or try to express himself in other words.

There is another component, however. I recommend slightly activist approach, selectively summing up the healthiest aspects of the person's angry, complex, multifaceted communication and statements. If you sum up a person's worst impulses, they will perceive that you are in agreement with what is most primitive and aggressive within them. If you sum up the healthy aspects of a patient's communication, you will direct them toward resolution and draw out the part of them that *does* wish to resolve the conflict. On the other hand, if they are bent on causing mayhem, they will correct you by escalating what they are saying, believing that you are not getting the message. After all, if they are angry and talking to you, they are trying to communicate with you.

Example: An over-the-top example of choosing what to sum up

Angry person: "I am so mad at my daughter that I could just wring her neck!"

1. Incorrect paraphrase: "You want to murder your daughter."
2. Correct paraphrase: "You are *really* furious with her!"

If you have, in the second example, accurately summed up the meaning of the angry person's image, they will go on to the next layer.

Angry person: "You will not believe what she did. I come home and find her on the couch lip-locking that punk from down the street. You know, the kid who epoxies his hair in corkscrew spikes?"

If, however, you are *inaccurate* in your summation of the second example, the other person will correct you with more vehemence.

Angry person: "No, not 'really upset.' I honestly want to loop a belt around her neck and strangle her. Seriously! She better not be home when I get back."

Lest there be any misunderstanding, in the second example, you have, through paraphrasing, revealed that the father actually does intend to commit homicide. Of course, your next step would be either very active verbal intervention to dissuade him from this action or calling the police. Or both.

Why a Paraphrase Instead of a Question?

More often than not, asking questions is not a good idea with really angry people, because questions demand answers. They are already using anger in an attempt to make you "get" what they are saying, and a question shows that you don't. This makes them try harder, usually with even more anger and less organization and coherence than before. They experience your questions as their failure to communicate, combining their anger with a sense of powerlessness and frustration. In this state of mind, the angry patient feels like they are in a fight, one that they are losing. In essence, they experience a question – a demand for an answer – as putting you in a dominant position.

Example: Questions can flame you up

To illustrate how even the simplest, most innocent question can lead to feelings of annoyance, irritation, or even an explosion of anger, consider the following.

Imagine coming home after a bad day; you are hot, tired, and frustrated. You walk into your house, drop your bags on the floor, sigh loudly, and walk toward the shower. Your spouse says, "Did you have a bad day?" Isn't this irritating? Isn't it *obvious* you've had a bad day? After all these years together, he or she doesn't know when a bad day just walked into the house!

On the other hand, imagine your spouse observes you and says, "Bad day, huh?" You don't have to explain anything. You continue walking toward the shower and say, "I don't want to talk now. I just want to take a shower. I'll talk to you later." You are not "forced" to explain yourself or provide an answer.

Layers of Anger

One useful image to associate with anger is an onion: layer upon layer. All that shows, however, is the top layer. You may think you know what is inside: "I know what you are really upset about. It is not about her standing you up on the date. This is really about your marriage breaking up, isn't it? Your husband left you too." However, the angry person did not solicit your invasive "wisdom": such a statement is an outrageous taking of liberties even if you are right. Furthermore, the underlying layers of the person's anger, and more centrally, character, are unpredictable. Not only will you be wrong even when you are "right," but you will also, very often, be wrong altogether.

However, when you properly use paraphrasing, you sum up in a phrase or sentence what the person has just said in a paragraph. If you paraphrase accurately, you've established that you've "gotten" it that far, so that the person does not have to repeat what they've said or try to say it in other words. It is like peeling off a single layer of that onion, so that you can see the next one. If you don't show that you "get" it, the person will feel compelled to repeat and/or elaborate that layer of the problem with more and more vehemence. The wonderful thing about paraphrasing is that you don't have to be "smart" and interpret anything. You simply have to listen carefully, layer by layer, until you reach the core level that is driving their anger. Frequently, this is their code of living (Chapter 43).

Example: Correct paraphrasing based on the "outrageous" example above (being stood up on a date, related to "abandonment" issues)

Shoshona: "I can't believe it. He is so stupid!"

You: "You are really upset!"

Shoshona: "Not upset. I'm furious!"

NOTE: *When you sum up imprecisely, the other person usually corrects you. This is as if she were tuning up the signal rather than arguing with you.*

You: "I haven't seen you this mad in a long time."

NOTE: *You can include extra information ("in a long time," for example). This is for the purpose of gently steering the person in a positive direction. It also helps to assess how responsive she is to you. In other words, if you add a little something, is she even able to hear it? In validating that she hasn't been angry in a long time, you are indicating that you are aware that she has shown that she is able to maintain control of herself.*

Shoshona: "I know. But nobody's ever done anything like this to me!"
You: "This is something new, huh?"

Shoshona: "Yeah, I asked him out last week, and he said yes, and then, in front of everybody, he said he was just joking."

You: "You must have been so embarrassed!"

Shoshona: "I was ashamed. It was just like when my husband left. I felt like I wasn't good enough for anybody."

NOTE: *Notice how Shoshona reveals the very thing we discussed above in the previous "outrageous" example. But she did it herself, because she voluntarily peeled off the intervening layers. And at each step, all you did was sum up what she said. Rather than feeling invaded, she offers you that deeply personal information willingly, as an act of trust.*

How to use paraphrasing successfully

- Your voice must be strong and firm, yet also calm. You speak to the person as someone who has the power to resolve the problem safely for all concerned, not as someone who is fragile or volatile (even if they are).

- You must contact the strong, positive aspects of the person, that which is striving for strength or simply looking for integrity. If you focus attention on the person's weaknesses and insecurities, you may foster behavior regression, which is often impulsive or violent. One of the easiest ways to encourage such regression is a soft, tender voice.
- Sometimes, you can use a dramatic paraphrase: "You are really ticked off!" Here, you sum up the individual's mood with your voice and posture, in addition to what they are saying.

Example: How I learned what not to do

I was interviewing an acutely suicidal fourteen-year-old girl in a detention facility. Several years previously, she had witnessed her mother murder her baby brother by breaking his spine over her knee. Furthermore, her mother was now manipulating her from prison, writing, "I didn't kill him, the alcohol did it. I've forgiven myself, and you have to forgive me too." The young girl told me that she had one wish: to commit a serious enough felony that she would be put in the same prison so that she could care for her mother. My heart breaking for her as she cried in front of me, I said softly and tenderly, "It's been really rough for you, huh?" She picked up her head, tears on her cheeks, and snarled, "Tell me something, do all you therapists learn to talk like that in school, or were you born that way?" In essence, she was saying, "I have just told you that I am bereft of a mother. I have no one to care for me. And you? How dare you come into my cell, a man I will never see again, and talk to me like you are going to be my new mother?" I put down my head a long moment, then looked in her eyes and said, "I'm sorry. Can we start over?" Beginning again was not easy. It took a long time before I could regain any trust from her, although eventually, we did establish enough rapport so that I could help her through her suicidal crisis.

What should I have said had I done things right? The problem wasn't my words – it was my tone of voice. Instead of speaking in a soft, gentle voice, I should have said, "It's been really rough for you," in a strong tone that expressed the following message: "Kid, this is a terrible situation. It's not fair, and it's not your fault, but let's not have any illusions, you and I. I can't save you. All I can offer you is a few tools to help you save yourself. It's up to you to pick them up."

By speaking with a strong voice, and not asking insipid questions, you are far less likely to further agitate the person, or cause them to stare at you in disbelief at the folly of your attempts to communicate. Remember, angry and agitated people are not looking for your sympathy. I have several times mentioned the oft-used word "respect." When we treat someone with respect, we are not trying to make them into something we'd like better, or reframe the situation in a way that would make us more comfortable. A true paraphrase pays respect to the person as he or she is.

Using Paraphrasing to Communicate with Severely Mentally Ill Individuals

Paraphrasing can be remarkably effective for communication with severely mentally ill people. Given the internal chaos that people experience when psychotic, manic or disorganized, it is essential that we do not add to their sense of confusion by barraging them with questions, or attempting to solve their problems by "taking over" and telling them what they should feel or do. Using paraphrasing, you can usually guide the mentally ill patient toward a state of mutual understanding, and an agreement that the immediate crisis needs to be resolved safely.

Example #1: Paraphrasing with a psychotic patient

Emily, about to give birth in the hospital, is in a midst of a psychotic episode. When the hospital social worker visited her to check if she'd signed a release of information, he found her in a decompensated state. She said, "There were pink rose petals, rose petals flying all around my head, clouds and clouds of roses." The social worker could have asked her a lot of questions in order to have her explain what she meant, but instead, he summed up the only thing he did grasp. (**NOTE**: This is not the *only* possible response. The social worker could have paraphrased another way; this is just one example.)

- Social worker: "Pretty confusing, huh?"
- Emily: "You are darn right it's confusing. How'd you like to be in my head?" *(This is the second layer of communication.)*
- Social worker: "I wouldn't want to be in a confused head. It must be hard to think."
- Emily: "Hard to think and scary. The roses spin and fly away, and I fly apart."
- Social worker: "You can't keep things together."
- Emily *(nodding)*: "I might fly to pieces, me and the baby."
- Social worker *(perceiving her affect, sums up what he believes to be her mood)*: "Pretty scary, huh?"
- Emily: "Yes, if the baby dies, I'll be apart forever."
- Social worker: "You are worried about the birth, huh?"

NOTE: *"Huh?" is not really a question; it is an invitation to the person to correct them if they are not fully accurate in their summation.*

- Emily: "Not worried. Terribly, terribly, terribly terrified."

Example #2: Paraphrasing with a treatment-resistant patient

Perry: "I never get enough sleep."

Nurse: "You look really tired."

Perry: "I don't know how I look, but I feel exhausted!"

When you are inaccurate in your summation, the other person usually corrects you. He is not arguing with you, just tuning up the signal.

Nurse: "You've been up late the last couple days, waking early, and now you are really tired, aren't you?"

You can include extra information that sums up the experience the other is having. This is for the purpose of slightly steering the person toward problem solving while not giving advice. It also allows you simply to assess how responsive the person is to you. In other words, if you add a little something, is he even able to hear it?

Perry: "I am not tired at night."

Nurse: "You can't fall asleep when you go to bed, huh?"

Notice the tag lines like, "huh?" or "aren't you?" These are not really questions. They follow statements and give the other person an <u>invitation</u> to correct you or give you more information.

Perry: "I don't even bother going to bed. I just lie there looking at the ceiling if I do."

Nurse: "It seems like a waste of time, and then you wake up early anyway. It'd be fine if you weren't tired."

This sentence by the nurse is an attempt to paraphrase what she believes are Perry's feelings about his sleep cycle. It is also another assessment: she offers Perry something to agree with or correct.

Perry: "Yeah. I'd be fine if I wasn't tired. I'd just sleep less and do more. But I'm too tired for that. I wonder if I need to talk to Dr. Montour about my medications. I think I need something to help me sleep."

Imagine that Perry is a young man who is very resistant to talking about his medications. If the nurse had immediately responded to his initial statement about being tired by suggesting he go to the doctor ("problem solving"), Perry might have angrily stopped talking or argued with her. By listening and showing step-by-step that she understood him, the nurse allowed Perry to find the "deeper layer" of his concern by himself.

Reaching the Core of the Problem

We know we have reached the core level of the person's problem when no more progress is being made. The person "spins his wheels", using different words, but essentially saying the same thing over and over again. On other occasions, they express relief at finally being understood, or exhibit an intensification of emotion, because you have reached that which is most distressing to them. When you reach core, and it is clear that you are on the same wavelength, <u>then</u> you can begin problem solving. Reaching the core problem can be achieved by the following:

- **Further validation**. You continue to show greater and greater understanding about their problem(s).
- **A summation of the core problem, followed by a puzzled "why?"** (**NOTE**: this "summing up why" is the only time that a "why" question is tactically sound.) For example, "You trusted him, and told him about the situation with your wife. He told the entire unit after you asked him to keep it secret. I can understand why you'd be so furious at him. What I am confused about is if you do break his arm, he wins. He gets hurt, sure, but you will go to jail. Given that this is the situation, why would you want to go after him instead of figuring out a way that you want really win, without getting in trouble?"
- **Establishing trust**. With some individuals, validation establishes you as a person of trust. In such cases, you can now be quite directive, because the patient is often willing to accept advice or instruction from people they trust.
- **Collaboration**. After reaching the core of the problem, the staff person and the patient can engage in a collaborative process of problem solving; trying to figure out a way to resolve the situation that is in the best interest of everyone involved.

"Socratic" Summation: Guiding Them to a Logical Conclusion

Here you guide the person to a logical conclusion. Imagine that each statement in the following sequence was preceded by a statement, perhaps one line, perhaps several paragraphs.

Example: Socratic summation

- So, let me make sure I got this straight. You think Dr. Glazer doesn't like you.
- You aren't sure, though, because he smiled at you.
- But you think maybe he doesn't like you because the meds upset your stomach, and you wonder if maybe he prescribed them to do that.
- You like the trip to his office across the campus here because it's so pretty by the river, and you wouldn't want to change to another doctor unless you had to.
- And you are telling me this because you want to figure out a way to work out this problem.
- You haven't been able to figure this out on your own, and it's making you really nervous and angry.
- You chose me because you trust me.

"So here's my idea. Since you trust me, how about you and I visit your doctor together, we can tell him about the upset stomach, *and if you think it's a good idea, you can ask him if he likes you or not. You can tell him why you are concerned, and I will be beside you so you won't have to worry that you will get in trouble for asking.*"

Notice that, through Socratic summation, you paint the person into a corner: actually, using their own logic, the person painted herself in a corner, and she "has to" accept your help, based on their own logic that you summed up.

Don't Waste It

While paraphrasing is a useful and necessary tool for de-escalation and communication with an angry person, this technique is too important to waste on everyday interactions. If your patients become used to you using paraphrasing as your primary method of discourse, they will soon become jaded, seeing it as a rather spiritless and irresolute response. It is "cold fare" compared to a rich dialogue, a combustible exchange of views, or a lush conversation. If your patients are calm, and are attempting find out what you think and who you are, be human in return! Simply talk with them.

However, if there is a crisis, and the individual does *not* believe they are understood, paraphrasing *now* comes into its own. It can have an almost electrifying effect on an angry person. Imagine the feeling of relief you get when trying to remove a splinter from under your fingernail, and after ten long minutes of aggravating struggle, you finally get a hold of it, and pull it out of your nail bed. That is the sense of relief that an angry patient, desperate to be heard, feels when they realize that the other person "gets it."

How to master paraphrasing

As you as you view paraphrasing as a 'specialized,' technique, you probably won't want to do it— and you won't be good at it anyway. When you are hit by adrenaline, dealing with an angry patient, perhaps in the throes of mental illness or intoxication, you will stumble over your words if you try to remember to say things like:

- "So what you are sharing with me is . . ."
- "What I hear you saying is . . ."

Don't do this! Many people will find you irritating, and you will be in your head at a time where you must be aware of what's going on in front of you.

You are, in fact, a master of paraphrasing. You do it all the time simply keeping a conversation going, saying things like:

- "Your kid flunked out, huh?"
- "You're not getting a raise."
- "You hate that guy."
- "She's the one."

In short, the natural statements you intersperse in any conversation are perfect paraphrasing. However, because you do this unconsciously, it's hard to tap into as an *emergency technique*. It's easy to perfect, however. Consider this—how many conversations do you have a day? Twenty? Thirty?

Forty? <u>In each and every conversation, at an arbitrary moment of your choosing, decide to paraphrase the next thing they say.</u> Just once. Your conversational partner won't even notice. But because you made a conscious decision to do this, your brain notices. That means you have practiced that skill twenty to forty times a day. Consider how good your skill at any physical activity would be if you do twenty, thirty, forty perfect repetitions every day—it would become automatic! Similarly, if you do this every day, you will be able to step into crisis oriented paraphrasing without hesitation. It will be so natural to you that you do not even have to think about it.

CHAPTER 45

Guidelines for
Limit Setting

Sometimes you have to draw a line. Once you have done this, however, it will become the main focus of your interchange. Therefore, do not ever set a limit that you can't enforce, or one that is not reasonable and simple to understand. Whenever possible, give the person time and space to make a choice. This also includes time for them (and you) to formulate a graceful way of disengaging.

Limit setting is often a kindness rather than oppression. Many people involved with hospital personnel are people whose lives are in chaos. Beleaguered by mental illness, struggling with substance abuse, beaten down by poverty or unemployment, such people experience their lives fragmenting into pieces. When the rules shift, they can become profoundly anxious.

Other people, more calculating, unilaterally change the rules through the application of such tactics as pure intimidation or passive-aggressive manipulation. This hurts all patients in the hospital; even the manipulative person loses. If the rules are fair and enforced with clarity and strength, our patients will also become clearer and stronger. Consider limits similar to the stakes we tie to a sapling, so that it grows straight and robust. It is when you know *where* you stand that you can actually gather your resources to stand on your own.

You must tell your patients what the rules are, and then ensure that they comply. Simply state what is required, or on other occasions, offer two choices, either one of which is acceptable to you. Then withdraw yourself from the exchange so that they have time to think.

There are times when you should physically withdraw. Don't be impatient. Offer a choice and "withdraw." Go to another room, if you can, so the person has time to think.

Other times, you simply withdraw from the debate itself, without leaving the patient's presence. Let us say that you set a limit, but the patient continues to try to argue with you. Your reply should be something like this: "I do understand you are upset, but there is nothing more to debate about the subject of shouting. The only thing you have to decide is this. You can lower your voice so that we *can* continue to discuss the problem, or we can end this for now and talk about it again another time."

Try to give the patient a face-saving way to disengage. In other words, if they do agree to the limit, they should feel that they are getting something for doing so. This is not a bribe, however. An example would be when the person says, "OK, I'll sit down. I will stop yelling. But now we'll talk about my boots, right?"

When setting a limit, your tone of voice should be matter-of-fact. You should not scold the other person or criticize them. Simply remind them of the rule or set a proper limit (a new rule, so to speak – something that may have been implicit, but has not been clearly enunciated).

Rules should be fair. They should also be possible for the patient to do: otherwise, it is a setup for failure. If you cannot clearly explain why the limit is necessary, at least to your peers, then it's not a good limit. One limit that is often very important to reiterate is the "social contract," such as, "We can work this out. But you know and I know one important thing: nobody is allowed to fight in this hospital. Nobody is allowed to hurt anybody here. We will talk things through and figure it out."

CHAPTER 46

Techniques that Don't Work
(or the Big Mistakes that Seemed
like Such Good Ideas)

Interacting with an angry individual can be intense, even frightening, if you are not both mentally and physically prepared. De-escalation requires on-the-scene improvisation, often with volatile and unpredictable people. In such a highly charged atmosphere, where clear communication is necessary to prevent any misunderstandings that may worsen the situation, you must be able to think quickly, but calmly, before speaking. By maintaining a professional emotional distance, and not reacting personally to anything the aggressor may say, you will be less likely to escalate an already heated situation.

That's the ideal. We all are less than perfect, however. Many mistakes are very obvious, and the moment something leaves our mouths we think, "Uh-oh. I shouldn't have said that!" Fortunately, you can prevent mistakes by taking a moment to gather your thoughts before responding to the aggressor. Sometimes you can hold up a hand to give them pause, gather your own resources, and then reply.

Some mistakes are subtler. On certain days, you may be tired, not feeling well, or distracted by family matters, and de-escalating an angry patient is the last thing you wish to do. Not surprisingly, risk increases when you are at less than your optimum ability and awareness.

The following topics are areas you should note to avoid making a blunder that leads to an escalating encounter with an angry person.

Do not try to ingratiate yourself with an angry person; do not pretend that a potentially aggressive situation or encounter has not developed by continuing to engage with them as you would normally; and, do not ignore the aggressive behavior or language while calmly going about your business in the hopes that they will eventually tire out. It can be very scary dealing with a threatening individual. At other times, we are just tired – we just don't have the energy to continue the argument, or we are sick of the subject, and we give in, letting the person have what they say they want, hoping that this will end the dispute.

Other professionals fool themselves. They let their patients vent feelings, making everyone in the milieu uncomfortable, but they try to tell themselves and others that they are just helping the person "express their emotions." In short, such people cover their eyes and hope for the best. One of the paradoxes of ingratiation is that staff who belie their professional integrity by allowing the aggressor to control their interactions often present themselves as having a "special rapport" with an aggressive patient who, in fact, intimidates them. Oddly enough, these same staff members, who try to avoid conflict, or "make nice," often suppress a lot of anger at being controlled by the person who frightens them. They displace this on those who call them on what they are doing. Thus, one of the first signs that the staff person is ingratiating him- or herself is often an attitude of self-righteousness, a defense mechanism that enables one to avoid questioning the violations of one's own integrity. The following factors are also signs of ingratiation:

- You worry about "how things are going" between yourself and the patient, and act or react accordingly. In particular, you worry if you are saying or doing the right things to make the person happy, calm, approving, etc.
- You are sometimes ashamed of your actions, or believe that you act cowardly when you interact with the patient.
- You believe you are caring and nice, so you react with shocked outrage when a patient is unkind, cruel, or aggressive toward you, as if you and the patient had made some sort of transaction that they have now betrayed.
- You allow the other to speak to you in overly familiar or rude terms, such as dude, buddy, pal, babe, or sweetheart. Do not ignore this. For example, you could say, "Michael, I'm your doctor. Don't call me 'dude.' I don't like that. I would like you to speak to me with the same respect that I speak to you."

Do not let the abnormal become normal. Consultation can be invaluable when you are concerned about an individual – or when you *should* be concerned and are not. Some professionals become so familiar with pathology that the abnormal becomes normal. The clinician no longer reacts in a natural way, tolerating or not noticing covert aggression, boundary trespass, or grooming behavior.

For others, even thinking about being in danger is so aversive that they blind themselves to boundary trespass, manipulation, or even blatant threats. A consultant may provide a fresh, hard-eyed perspective that shakes people out of a "trance of well-being," which is as illusory as a mouse sitting quietly in front of a snake, unaware of the danger because the snake is moving so easily and slowly.

Example: When the abnormal becomes normal

One client would approach staff with a smile and give them a bone-crushing hug, effusing how much she loved them. Staff both unsettled and physically hurt would firmly tell her to stop. However, because there was no general consultation that would have revealed these behaviors as "practice runs" for an assault, other staff were similarly grabbed. They had no plan to deal with her – everyone was on their own. Some fended her off, some tried to stop her verbally when she came close, and others tolerated the forceful embraces. One day the "hug" turned into a tackle and several staff were seriously hurt.

Do not make the mistake of mind reading. Sometimes, staff will try to connect with a potentially aggressive person by telling them how they must feel, by confessing to having the same issues, or claiming to have gone through a similar situation. As noted elsewhere, personal comparisons normally make the patient even more indignant at your assumed familiarity. Statements like, "I know how you feel," or "I know you love your son," or "When I . . ." are statements that the angry patient may not agree with at all.

When you make such a generalized statement, people may feel compelled to prove you wrong by doing or saying exactly the opposite. If you do want to say something positive, praise a specific action and say it like this, "I know you are really mad, so I really appreciate how hard you are trying to not yell." And of course, only praise them for something that is true.

Do not talk over the person. Being "professional" does not mean talking in jargon. Remember, people can feel trapped by words, and quite frequently, a health or social services person talks to the patient using vocabulary or explaining concepts that confirm a low sense of self-worth: "Gosh, he's been so nice, and explained things in such detail, but I cannot figure out what he is saying." In other cases, the patient or family experiences your elaborate sentences, arcane vocabulary, and barrage of acronyms as condescending. Do not, therefore, be "smarter" than your patient: your brilliant insights are often experienced as off the mark, confusing, or invasive.

Another dreadfully insulting type of talking over the patient is talking to family members or to professionals as if the patient is either an object or mentally incompetent to understand what you are saying.

Beware the dangers of venting. Venting is different from the situation described in Chapter 42 where you let someone "get something off their chest." In this case, the person has something that they have to say aloud: a complaint, a shameful secret, or a lot of frustration.

Venting is somewhat different, a kind of verbal aggression at one remove. Many people have a false idea about aggression, imagining it to be some kind of psychological fluid that builds up pressure inside of us. When we vent (hence the word), these people believe that we get rid of the anger and then become peaceful, similar to a valve releasing pressure from a water line. Aggression, however, is not a fluid; it is state of arousal. Just like any other state of arousal – sexuality, happiness, excited interest – additional stimuli elicits more arousal. When one shouts, yells, complains, kicks, or the like, one is stimulating oneself to greater and greater aggression. Therefore, if you allow a patient to vent angrily, the more aroused, and hence, dangerous they become. This only makes de-escalation more difficult.

Do not parse any distinctions between venting directed at other people, and either anger or rage. Simply consider it for what it is – aggression. When you let an angry person vent about other people, they perceive that you are giving implicit approval to their verbal complaints and abuse; they believe you are on their side. If you listen to their venting silently, without de-escalating or controlling their verbal escalation, they see it as a form of alliance or approval. However, when they get so angry that they start to become dangerous and *then* you object, they will turn on you, feeling betrayed. Thus, if an angry person begins to vent, de-escalate and control them.

Nod once or twice. In western culture, we generally nod our head once or twice followed by an interval of immobility while we listen to the other person. If we nod our head more than twice – particularly in rapid succession, this means we are not interested and wish the person would be silent. In some cultures, Japan being a prominent example, rapid and almost continuous head nodding and brief interjections like, "really, really, imagine that, yes, yes . . ." denotes interest. In other cultures, nodding while someone is talking is considered rude, and people will, instead, hold their head still and look directly at you as a sign of respect. It is examples like this that illustrate the necessity of "cultural information training." Nonetheless, if you wish to be perceived as truly listening with interest to someone in mainstream American culture, nod once or twice.

Reframe. Reframing is a therapeutic technique in which we attempt to help the other person perceive their situation from another perspective – a less negative perspective. For example, Johnny Cash's famous song, "A Boy Named Sue," is the story of a man who is forced to grow up tough because his father names him Sue, shortly before abandoning the family. The "reframe" is that his father did it for his own good, because in such a hard world, without a father's guidance and protection, this name served to make him strong enough to handle anything. You must be very cautious with reframing, because it can serve to trivialize the other's experience. A clinician who comments, "Consider you husband leaving you as a learning experience," or uses wishful thinking doesn't want to accept the full misery and terror of the other's situation. One example of the latter is to *impose* the appellation of "survivor" on a victim of rape or abuse. The <u>victim </u>deserves and needs a presence of someone who can face horror head on, standing beside them, not someone who tries to make it more palatable. It is often only when a person can accept the full implications of their victimization that they can begin to figure out how to survive. <u>Reframing, done incorrectly, can outrage the patient as they feel betrayed by the clinician undermining their perception of what happened to them.</u>

Avoid pushing forgiveness in the face of evil. Another therapeutic violation is an ideology that victims of evil can only heal when they forgive their violator. It is certainly true that some people come to this realization. Others never do, and many never should.[27] It is the therapeutic task to help the individual face what was done to them and what they have become. Further, it is to help them become as strong and resilient as possible, given the circumstances. It is certainly fine if they, on their own, begin to consider the implications of forgiving their attacker. A suggestion that they *should* on the part of the therapist or other social services person can truly outrage them, even driving them right out of treatment.

Do not become a chameleon. Do not try to create rapport with a person from another culture, including street and youth culture, by affecting slang that you have not lived. To be sure, some slang expressions are generic, but you can easily lose your professionalism if you speak too casually. When you further use slang that is specific to a culture that you are not part of, you will sound unnatural, as you will surely use some expressions that are out of date or out of context. To the recipient, you will seem either a fool or a suck-up.

Other Really Obvious Mistakes that We Shouldn't Do, But We Do Anyway

Although some of the items included in the following list have been discussed elsewhere in this book, they are repeated here to remind you of the seemingly minor, yet crucial, details of de-escalation. You should NOT do the following:

- Make promises you can't keep. This will be experienced as betrayal. If the angry person is already aware that you cannot enforce a consequence, or keep a promise, you will have damaged your credibility, perhaps irrevocably.
- Bombard them with choices, questions, and solutions, as this will only overwhelm the patient, especially if they are suffering from mental illness.
- Ask the upset person "why?" Asking a "why" question demands an answer or an explanation from the angry person, something they may be quite unwilling, or unable, to do. "Why" questions should only be used when you have used paraphrasing to reach the core problem successfully (see Chapter 44).
- Talk down to people as if they are stupid. Do not use unfamiliar vocabulary, jargon, or acronyms. Do not roll your eyes or sigh heavily while the patient is trying to communicate with you. Do not interrupt as they speak, particularly to correct what they are saying. On the other hand, interruption of aggressive verbalizations or pointless monologues on the part of the aggressive person IS the right thing to do.
- Speak to them as if they are fragile.
- Use global phrases like "calm down." Do not use "social services scolding" like "That's not appropriate." Phrases like this color you as someone uncomfortable in confronting aggression head on.
- Analyze why they do something. Analyzing is "cutting apart to examine." People, particularly upset or angered people, experience someone analyzing them not as a mark of the analyst's brilliance, but as a violation.
- Expose their private information in front of others.

Warning: Be careful of "hallway consultations"

You may be talking about a patient, either fully professionally, or in some cases, blowing off steam with complaints, jokes, or the like, and another individual hears you. That it is not them that you are talking about is irrelevant. They think, "If they talk about that woman, they are probably talking about me the same way. The thought of my nurse talking about my family with that smile on his face is intolerable!"

- Take things personally when the angry person attacks your character or professionalism. A measure of a true professional is NOT taking things personally.

- Allow the angry person to trespass on your personal boundaries. When we allow others to trespass upon us, we are, implicitly giving them permission. Any territory we relinquish is free to whoever chooses to occupy it.

- Suspend boundaries. If we become too familiar or friendly, we become "friends." Sharing personal information, or not setting limits in hopes that in so doing you will have better rapport with intimidating or difficult patients, leads the patient to view the relationship between you as eye-to-eye and reciprocal. It is very difficult to accept authority – limit setting, directions, or commands – from a friend or equal. Safety is enhanced when one enforces a respectful but real hierarchical relationship.

- Touch, push, or try to move them from one place to another with your hands, or point at them.

- Adopt an authoritarian or demeaning attitude, particularly in front of their peers. Authoritarian attitudes and behaviors are one of the most common precipitants of assault by patients.

CHAPTER 47

Enforcing Limits or Commands
When You Have Both Unquestionable
Authority and the Means to Enforce It

This section is specific to staff in an inpatient psychiatric hospital or group home, and for security officers in an agency. Use these strategies in emergency situations, when people are on the edge of aggression or another serious transgression.

Give clear directives with no wiggle room. For example, say in a confident, commanding voice, "Billy Jo, you are yelling too loudly. You have to go to your room."

If they do not comply with the directive, depersonalize the reiteration. "Billy Jo, you are required to go to your room. " Do NOT say, "I expect you to . . ." The individual should experience what you are saying as the "law," an institutional command or policy, rather than a personal issue between the two of you.

Don't get caught up in manipulative word games. Do not respond to professed ignorance or confusion. You are using this tactic because there is no ambiguity regarding the transgression, and no ambiguity what the consequence will be.

Give consequences. "If you do not go to your room, then . . ." Give the person the consequence. (Here a patient might be told that they will be escorted to their room, put in restraints, be suspended from a program, or asked to leave.)

Follow up with the "choice." This follows almost directly after the previous step. With a detached tone, you will say something like this: "It looks like you've got a decision to make." Followed by, conceivably, something like, "You're right. You don't have to voluntarily go to your room. Of course, you can do it, and relax there in peace. But if you choose not to, you know what will happen next. That's why I say that it looks like you have a choice to make." At this point, you can _slightly_ break eye contact, as if you are out of the game and the choice is in their hands.

<u>**Take action**</u>. If the person does not comply, you immediately enforce compliance, depending, on the circumstances and your authority.

SECTION VIII

Communication with
Mentally Ill and Emotionally
Disturbed Youth

CHAPTER 48

Working with Potentially
Aggressive Youth

De-escalation of Youth: Are There Any Differences from that of Adults?

Everyone desires to be respected and viewed as a mature, knowledgeable, and responsible person. Young people have a passionate desire for individuals worth respecting in their own lives. However, when children emerge into modern teenage society, they are not *primarily* concerned with either maturity or integrity as an adult, or security and happiness at home as a child. They desire to feel powerful and independent, and above all they desire respect. They measure power by their effect on others, particularly their peers. Many teens regard intimidation (ranging from actual acts of violence to such passive-aggressive acts as the "silent treatment," where a sullen teenager makes an adult anxious and overeager to reach them) as a means of achieving a powerful role in this world.

Teenagers, especially, experience fear and rage as being out of control. At the same time, they'd like to believe that through aggression they will *take* control. Every time you can deal firmly and effectively with an angry teenager without losing your temper, you demonstrate a kind of power that is at variance to loss of control. This is contained power, power expressed with dignity and grace, and it is very attractive to teens who may have never seen it before.

In this section, I will describe the character traits that are often related to aggression in youth, traits that express their fundamental attitude toward the world. View each chapter as a quick step-by-step process for establishing which mode of aggression younger patients are expressing, and strategies for de-escalation. Should one approach seem ineffective, move on to the next. Once you are aware of their characteristic style of aggression, start with that pattern as your default mode the next time he or she becomes aggressive.[28]

The general principles of de-escalation are the same for youth and adults

Generally speaking, you will use the same de-escalation strategies with youth that you do for adults (as described in this book). The differences are often more on nuance than on major details. I have, however, "subdivided" youth in some general categories based on behavior that will help you understand young people and use the best strategies to help stabilize and calm them when they become aggressive or are otherwise in crisis. As in other sections of the book, these categories are largely independent of diagnosis.

CHAPTER 49

No Brake Pads:
A Consideration of the
Impulsive Child

Children in the United States have been allegedly plagued by an epidemic of attention deficit disorder (ADD)/attention deficit hyperactivity disorder (ADHD). Per orthodox theory, attention disorders come in two major forms. In the first type, the main manifestation is a short attention span. In the second type, hyperactivity is also present. Although beyond the scope of this book, the diagnosis of ADD/ADHD, now so common, deserves more debate than it is currently receiving in both media and clinical sources.[29]

In any event, let us here consider the impulsive youth, one who tends to act before he or she thinks.

- He is in your emergency room and sees that a person has put down their pen on the chair and gotten up to speak with a nurse. Without considering the consequences, he steals it, right in front of the security camera.
- She gets in an argument with her fourteen-year-old, painfully shy sister, and blurts out something embarrassing about her body to her sister's new boyfriend.
- Another boy bumps him in the hall and he stabs him in the hand with his pencil: he is as surprised as the victim, both of them looking at the bloody pencil tip with their mouths open in shock.

Due to their difficulty in deriving satisfaction by methodical step-by-step work, as opposed to the thrill of immediate gratification, many impulsive youth engage in disruptive or thrill-seeking behaviors. Beyond any interventions, from educational and vocational planning to cognitive therapy or medication, the impulsive youth needs an activity that consumes their interest. They are able to focus with remarkable intensity when something fascinates them, about which they can say, "This is me." This activity gives purpose and meaning to their lives, a touchstone they can use to help them manage those more difficult situations where they do not feel at home.

The impulsive young person gets angry or aggressive for the same reasons that any other person would, but they get particularly upset and frustrated when someone interferes with the gratification of an impulse. Swept away by this anger, they find it difficult to stop themselves. Impulsive youths hear very little of what you say, particularly when they are angry, upset, or confused. Paraphrasing (see Chapter 44) is particularly valuable, as you prove that you understand their desire and frustration, rather than argue with them.

Impulsive youth track very little of what you say – particularly when they are very angry. If they are too escalated for paraphrasing, it is not the time for explanations, attempts to elicit empathy for the other person, or moral preachments. What is usually best is a calm demeanor and simple short commands.

Review: Dealing with the impulsive youth

When dealing with an upset or aggressive youth, assume that he or she is in "impulsive" mode until proven otherwise. How do you know that they are *not* merely impulsive or upset? If the strategies suitable for de-escalating an impulsive youth don't work, go on to the next strategy. Remember, we are talking about an approach that takes only a few moments – this is NOT a counseling session!

- Paraphrase.
- Give them firm, brief commands; help them regain control by directly telling them what to do.

CHAPTER 50

Conduct Disorder:
Fierce Youth

What is conduct disorder?

Conduct disorder is a term/diagnosis that delineates behaviors in children and youth that in someone over the age of eighteen would merit the diagnosis of antisocial personality disorder, or even psychopathy. However, because the child/adolescent brain is still so mutable, we properly do not give them a diagnosis that indicates that change is unlikely, if not impossible. The majority of children who fully merit the diagnosis of conduct disorder do NOT grow up to be psychopaths. Nonetheless, Chapters 12 and 13 on manipulation and psychopathy are essential in considering any youth who is conduct disordered because their behaviors, even if not fixed throughout the span of their lives, are currently the same. This section focuses specifically on youth who display ferocious, manipulative, or predatory behaviors, whatever the cause may be.

This is a disorder of childhood and teen years, and is often, though not definitively, a precursor of criminality, even psychopathy. Such youth often seem to be without conscience or caring for most other children or adults.

The conduct-disordered youth typically displays rages in three major categories: fury, aggressive-manipulative, and predatory behavior (Section IX). Conduct-disordered character traits can develop from a myriad of reasons, some of them heart-rending. This is relevant in future treatment, but not for the de-escalation and control of their anger or violence. Particularly with these fierce young people, someone will be seriously hurt if you contextualize or excuse their behavior.

Attempting to establish a sympathetic or nurturing connection with an aggressive young person is often a mistake, particularly during a rage state, and this is *particularly* true with such fierce youth. They experience these gestures as an attempt to soften their defenses, and/or as a sign of weakness on your part. In other words, sympathy is experienced as manipulation or an attack. Fierce youth, with their poor ability to form attachments, lay extreme importance on protecting themselves from "invasion." Thus, any loss of control, which is implicit in a softened response, is viewed as weakness.

They strive to defend themselves against any emotional need or attachments with others by building up a callous attitude, one without sympathy for or even understanding of other people's pain. In the most basic and existential sense, such youth are profoundly isolated, without human ties. They are left with an inflated and easily bruised sense of pride and respect, their most important "possessions," something for which they will live and die. This pride, however, can be an access route for communication and de-escalation. The formula for communication with such fierce youth is "respect outweighs sympathy."

In other words, enforce the rules with calm gravity and strength, and never try to ingratiate yourself, as this will invite contempt. Similarly, trying to "prove" that you care will have a negative effect. If you manifest yourself as a strong and dignified professional who does not make it "personal" when you give advice or set limits, you will, sometimes draw their attention and curiosity. The youth might begin to question: "How come she has nothing to prove? Why, even though she isn't frightening or even trying to frighten me, is she not weak? Why isn't she, like so many others, sucking up to me, trying to please me?" If there is hope for such youth, it lies in their fascination with power. You present to them a world unimaginable, one where power and human decency can exist within the same body. If you do not behave in this manner yourself, such a fierce young person will be unreachable.

Review: Dealing with conduct-disordered (fierce) youth

You first approached the youth as if their aggression is impulsive and you tried to exert authority of them. That didn't work – instead, the youth becomes more focused and directed in his or her aggression toward you.

- Let them know where they stand, that anything you are requiring isn't "personal," you are just doing your job.
- Dispassionately enforce your authority. Deal with them on a professional, slightly disinterested basis.
- Respect before sympathy! Don't try to *prove* you care.

CHAPTER 51

Dynamite under a Rock:
Explosive Youth

The hallmark quality of these young patients is that once their fiery temper is unleashed, it is very hard for them to stop. They rage and rage. Despite their explosive personality, many of these younger patients do not necessarily have attention or impulse problems, and they can pay attention when they choose to do so. Others, such as the child with fetal alcohol spectrum disorders, or a history of head injuries, cannot pay attention very well in the best of circumstances, in addition to their explosive tempers. Regardless, they are the kids of whom one says in a unit staff meeting, "Billy lost it again today," and everyone nods, imagining the slung chairs, classroom supplies, and the young person raging for over an hour *after* they were restrained on a gurney or in a quiet room.

Orders or even firm commands do not work well with these young people. In fact, they may view such commands as further provocation, heightening their anger instead of calming them. The watchword, instead, is containment. You *will* give commands, but your voice must be firm and calm, even quiet. The command is to get their attention to focus everything on one being – you. In favorable circumstances, you, and however many staff are necessary, can escort this young person to a quiet area where they calm down on their own. Your task is to monitor them so that they do not injure themselves or damage property. You cannot, however, problem solve or otherwise work things out while they are still on fire. If you are unable to do this, you should avail yourself of the strategies in Section IX, particularly Chapter 59 on hot rage.

Children with neurological deficits

Some such youth, particularly those with neurological damage, will also suddenly shift into an "organic rage," apparently unmediated by cognitive processes. However, these kids often show small micro-changes of behavior right before assaults. With youth with whom you have an ongoing relationship, you should definitely do what you can to learn these signs to help them shift gears into another activity or process, thereby heading off the explosion. This is something you should raise with the youth's treatment professionals as well.

- A girl in a group home had enacted a number of apparently sudden severe attacks against other residents. We found that when she focused on an intellectual task too long, she would begin scratching at her forearm. The "sudden" explosion of aggression followed a few minutes after this "tell."
- Another youth would knit his brows and glower in a stubborn manner when he didn't understand a conversation. He interpreted this as people "making me feel stupid," an attack in his view. This facial expression was a clear sign to slow down, lighten up, or change the subject.

Review: Dealing with explosive youth

You attempted to exert authority on an aggressive youth, and then, when that didn't work, you used the professional respect, command presence and distance that are best with the fierce youth. When the youth continues to ramp upward into further aggression, assume you are dealing with an explosive youth. They get more and more aggressive without a "circuit breaker" that helps them turn off. They become very reactive to just about anything you say or do.

- Rage is usually explosive. They often have no fear of harm when in an explosive rage state.
- Don't get flamed up yourself, no matter what they say (which will frequently be pretty bad!).
- If you speak at all, use paraphrasing (see Chapter 43). The explosive youth, however, will often react with more rage even to paraphrasing. In their rage, they view paraphrasing as mocking them.
- Silently, implacably, take them somewhere safe, where they are contained and unable to harm anything. Wait them out.

CHAPTER 52

"Even if You Make Me, I'll Still Make You Miserable": Opposition-defiant Kids

Oppositional-defiant disorder (ODD) is considered a behavioral disorder of childhood. ODD usually develops with upbringing typified by poor boundaries (too invasive, too lax, or both). Aggression is typically against family members and those familiar to the child. Dictatorial parents, in an effort to "break" the child to their will, often "create" ODD youth among those who are too strong-willed to submit. The ODD kid's motto seems to be, "You will not break me. Furthermore, even if you make me do it, I still say no." Parents who are not consistent or who do not enforce reasonable discipline, being either overly permissive or chaotic, also elicit such behaviors. In this case, the child is implicitly saying, "I will act out until you are forced to give me some limits."

In many cases, however, the parents have not raised their children poorly, but their child has bonded with other poorly disciplined children, or they may be trying to imitate behaviors they absorbed from television, movies, or video games. Furthermore, experimental drug or alcohol use, and subsequent abuse, can easily transform a well-behaved and respectful youth into an oppositional and defiant one.

Negative reinforcement – primarily giving attention for negative behavior – will elicit more negative behaviors. Reinforcement through punishment that is both out of proportion or inconsistent teaches the child that discipline is an attack, that the parent or staff person is unpredictable, and that acting out at least garners parental attention. In their own way, these youth have discovered that their defiant behaviors give them a sense of power over adults, be they parents, teachers, or hospital staff, because they know they can get a reaction, even if that reaction is punishment. Once power is acquired in this manner, the youth adopts a grandiose sense of importance, and frustrating and defying adults becomes its own reward.

Oppositional-defiant youth are surpassingly argumentative, fighting over fine points, while claiming to be misunderstood. They apparently thrive on conflict, and they look for any pretext to continue the argument. Such behavior is not a search for truth or understanding: it is simply a power tactic. They actually hold in contempt adults who take this overly seriously but feel compelled to test over-and-over again if you are worthy of respect. If you are losing your temper, they are winning. This need to argue, at its extreme end, seems related to obsessive-compulsive disorder; their brain, apparently, will not let go of their place in the argument. Right and wrong do not matter; only their definition of "right" at the moment matters. Although ODD youth can sometimes be violent, their aggression seems engendered by resistance to authority and perhaps an unconscious desire that a clear, trustworthy, and consistent authority be exerted over them so that their place in the world is well defined. The oppositional youth will test these boundaries over and over again to see if the limits have changed.

The watchword in dealing with these kids is to pick your battles. Do not waste energy arguing about anything that is not important. When it is important, become implacable. They put energy in their argument, you respond with a calm, yet unwavering resolve. As an adult, you should never argue with such a youth as an "equal"; instead, tell them what will be, with no negotiation whatsoever. If you are correct in what you require, it should be experienced as a force like gravity – not a debate.

These youth are used to a lot of attention when they argue or resist. Because this drains so much energy from those responsible for them, they are often ignored when they are not making trouble, much less acting positively. Therefore, be sure to notice when they are acting with integrity, agreeableness, or respect, so that they experience positive attention for these actions.

Review: Dealing with oppositional-defiant kids

These young people argue for argument's sake. Their reward is the negative attention they require from adults, and the sense that they have you – at least your moods – under their control. They believe they've won if they anger you or make you upset.

- Pick your battles. Disengage from those not worth arguing.
- If it is an issue worth confronting, require them to follow your instructions. Be like a force as unyielding as gravity – there is no argument with that.
- Whenever possible, give extra energy (positive attention) to the young person who is doing something worthwhile or worth respecting.

CHAPTER 53

PTSD in
Young People

For both children and youth, post-traumatic stress disorder, including either the experience or the witnessing of severe violence, is often physically enacted rather than verbalized. Young men in particular, who would adamantly deny ever experiencing trauma, seem to live by Nietzsche's adage, "that which does not kill me makes me stronger."

There is no unique de-escalation method for use with traumatized youth, as they can display aggression and violence in a variety of modes, from terrified and chaotic rage to purposeful predation. However, their violence is essential clinical data. If you were to examine any aggressive or violent episode by such a youth, you will have, in symbolic form, the story of their own trauma, not only what happened to them, but also what was created *within* them. Traumatized children, in particular, often display terrified rage (Chapter 58). The more predatory or furious rage that some children and teenagers exhibit is a kind of reaction formation; they have found a way to cease experiencing the pervasive dread of the victim. Tragically, however, this often results in their only feeling safe in the role of the victimizer.

Circular breathing (Chapter 24) contains a method that you can, on occasion, teach to traumatized youth that can help them turn trauma ("lived experience") into memory ("past experience"). Circular breathing is particularly useful with those who are guarded against both therapy and help from others, because it is a do-it-yourself procedure, which allows them to feel in control. You can, quite honestly, introduce it as a martial arts technique to control the mind rather than as a therapy method – the latter being something the youth may resist.[30]

CHAPTER 54

Pseudo-nihilism

By definition, nihilism means a general rejection of customary beliefs, and the belief that there is no meaning or purpose in existence. Such a youth, who may affect a posture that includes ennui, self-destructive behaviors, or affected disinterest, is, in fact, striving for power. Juveniles who adopt this outlook feel a sense of control when they horrify, disgust, or offend others. Nihilistic youths may also display an aloof callousness, with a distinct lack of sympathy for the feelings and emotions of others. By making themselves outcasts, they are inviolate vis-à-vis the larger society and its goals.

When interacting with these young people, you should not be emotionally bland, distant, or apathetic. Instead, pay attention to what the youth presents and offer them a human reaction. If you try to make yourself impervious, pretending that their provocative behaviors do not affect you, they may escalate until they do evoke a reaction. If you do succeed in "stonewalling" them, all you have succeeded in doing is establishing that you, like they, don't care.

Despite their outwardly indifferent attitude and persona, these young patients are in need of an adult to be a *fair witness* to their world, able to provide feedback in a way that he or she does not feel compelled to resist. They need to talk with someone with more life experience, someone who is not going to abuse them, abandon them, or treat them unfairly. At the same time, do not imagine this as a heart-to-heart discussion, facing each other, with the youth "opening up" to your unconditional positive regard. You are far more likely trusted when you do not try so hard – when you sit side by side, with only occasional eye contact. You must be neither detached nor eager. By being at ease, you manifest a state of being that these young people crave above all else.

Review: Dealing with pseudo-nihilism

Not only may they be aggressive, but they may also be focused on NOT making a link with you, treating you with withdrawn or sullen indifference. Other youth may be very much at odds with you; they may even rage or curse at you. These kids try to cut themselves off from you.

1. Don't try to make them change or "feel better." They will regard "put ups" (and you) with contempt.
2. They may try to repel you with what they say, or say they have done. Give them a human reaction, but not an overreaction.
3. They are most dangerous when left alone to stew in their own juices. Be the adult that they almost surely do not have in their life, so that they have a moral touchstone.

CHAPTER 55

Therapeutic Communication
with Abused Children and Teens

This section is particularly relevant to those who work with abused children and teens. Be aware that therapy itself can evoke profound rage. The youth will experience therapy as further abuse if the clinician does not take into account the real needs of the child. This *therapeutic abuse,* particularly in regard to abused children, results where the theories, preconceptions, and anxieties of the therapist lead them to ignore what is really necessary for the child to recover and thrive. Please refer to the work of Anna Salter for more information on the points enumerated below.[31X]

Children who are abused by narcissistic people who never see them as they are – who tell the child, for example, "how much I love you, how I know you want to do this too: – often need a therapist who can see *into* them: see their heart, and make that manifest. Such a therapist is not "insight proud": their task is not to demonstrate to the child or youth how wise they are, but to pay exquisite attention, demonstrating to the child that they truly do perceive them as the child actually knows himself or herself to be.

The victim of sadistic abuse, physical or emotional, has suffered an excruciating examination of every nuance of movement and expression, because it is their suffering that gives the abuser pleasure. Such children feel flayed and exposed. The therapist must leave opening and revelation to the child. Even if you are right when you "go ahead of them," you will be traumatizing the child as you expose him or her to the cruelty of your insight.

Don't just sit and listen!

One of the most frequent complaints I have heard from teenagers about other therapists is that "they just sit there." Or, "All they do is repeat what I say." They also hate being treated as fragile, no matter how awful their lives have been. Even those children who seem to respond to the latter feel that they are selling themselves out – accepting a definition of themselves as fragile defines them as a victim, forever.

Children who have suffered abuse often go to therapy to find a new perspective, and through this, to define themselves anew. This can be either to discover new ways of experiencing the world, or to finally have an opportunity for their true self to emerge. When they are mirrored as fragile, this opportunity is taken from them. The world they live in is one they wish to leave, and one way to do so is to meet and establish a genuine dialogue with an adult who can facilitate an opportunity for them to open their eyes to new worlds.

SECTION IX

Managing Rage and Violence

CHAPTER 56

Preface to Rage

Rage and anger are not merely different in degree; they are different modes of being, just as water, once past the boiling point, becomes steam. Angry people posture to establish dominance or to force agreement or compliance from others. If nothing else, their goal is to communicate their feelings, although, due to their lack of interpersonal skills, their mental illness, or the effects of drugs and/or alcohol, they often resort to anger in an attempt to make themselves heard.

The reader will recall that anger is denoted as falling between 20 and 95 on the aggressiveness scale (Chapter 34). This represents a very broad range of arousal, ranging from mildly irritated to truly irate. Rage, however, occupies a much smaller fraction of the scale, from 95 to 99. An enraged person desires to commit mayhem. They are in a "threshold" state, their anger and rage escalating until they have overcome any moral or personal constraints that may prohibit them from committing the ultimate expression of rage – violence.

Taking into account that the numbers in the aggression scale are images rather than scientific measurements, you still may use some of the de-escalation for anger when, for example, the person is at 93. The tactic of "breaking the pattern" (Chapter 42) can be effective at just these moments; you can say something so unexpected that the fight just "drops out of the person." Past a certain point, however, their only focus is overcoming what is holding them back: fear of consequences, damage to their self-image, and innate morality. Their internal restraints are "fighting" a battle inside them with their primitive desire to maim and destroy. At this point, all the strategies for dealing with the angry person are more or less useless.

When we are facing an enraged person from whom we cannot escape, or our professional and moral responsibilities require us to stay, <u>our task is to control the situation *and* the other person so that their inhibitions are strengthened</u>. In this sense, what we refer to as "control" is actually supporting the best aspects of the enraged person until they are able, once again, to live in peace without that imposition of control.

Example: The power of internal restraints

As one man who had been in a manic psychosis told me half a year later, "You came into my room and I decided to kill you. I was just about to make my move, and a voice in my head said, 'You are not allowed to kill him. He's your friend.' I couldn't remember exactly what a friend was, but the voice said, 'I don't care if you remember. It's against the rules to kill your friends.'" Only aware of his hair-trigger tension, I left his room, perhaps saving my life in the process.

There are various types of rage. It is very important to recognize what type of rage the person is expressing, because we have different strategies to deal with each type. At the same time, do not worry that you will have a lot to remember. Enraged people's behavior is quite obvious – after reading this section, you will easily be able to tell what type of rage they are in, and will, therefore, know the best strategies to use to control them.[32]

IMPORTANT CAUTION

Here, and in several other areas of this book, I have used animal symbols to aid in the understanding of various types of rage or other behavior. For example, I use the image of a leopard or a shark in describing predatory rage. These are thought devices and are not intended to be used in either paperwork or communication to describe patients. In our hypersensitive times, such a reference to a specific patient may be misconstrued as stigmatizing them as "being an animal." Nothing could be further than the truth – the images are to assist in understanding modes of behavior, not character. Nonetheless, such images should remain aids of understanding, not terms of reference.

CHAPTER 57

Chaotic Rage: A Consideration
of Rage Emerging from
Various Disorganized States

Signs of Chaotic Rage

Disorganized individuals enter into chaotic rage states for many of the same reasons that prompt agitation and anger in anyone: frustration, fear, confusion caused by too much stimulation, and feelings of invasion (for example, when you must carry out a necessary medical task that they do not understand or that is physically disconcerting). Chaotic rage is typified by profound disorganization of cognitive and perceptual processes, and can be engendered by severe psychosis that has "crossed over" into a delirium state, mania, intoxication, drug withdrawal, severe intellectual/developmental disabilities, senile dementia, overwhelming emotions, or a result of brain injury or trauma. The individual is profoundly disoriented, often experiencing severe hallucinations, illusions, and delusional thinking.

Whatever the cause, chaotic rage requires a similar response

Lest there be any confusion, I am not asserting that such different syndromes as severe intellectual/developmental disabilities, senile dementia, intoxication, etc., are the same. I am, however, asserting that the manifestation of rage in a variety of people – chaotic rage, whatever the cause – requires a similar response.

Unlike a classic psychosis, the most salient characteristic is the near impossibility of establishing _any_ lines of communication with them. Individuals in this state often cannot logically string words together, communicating in ways that are comprehensible only to themselves. They may utter nonsensical cascades of words, grunts, moans, or mumblings. Others make sentences based on rhymes, puns, or cross-meanings, their brains capriciously linking words together based on sounds, not meanings. The delirious individual may laugh or babble without any clear object of mirth, or completely at variance to the seriousness of the situation. They may speak in repetitive loops, fixating on one subject, which could be real, delusional, or such a manifestation of their disorganization that you do not even know what they are talking about.

Patients in chaotic rage states can easily become quite frightened or irritable, especially if they are overwhelmed with stimuli, such as a group of onlookers. They may begin yelling, screaming, lashing out physically, engaging in such self-injurious acts as scratching and gouging their own flesh, striking themselves repeatedly, or banging their head against the wall or ground.

Their rage sometimes explodes, seemingly, out of nowhere. People in a chaotic rage state strike out in all directions: they are not coordinated, but they are disinhibited. What this means is that nothing, no fear of injury or consequences, holds them back from their attack. They may grab, scratch, bite, kick, and strike in flailing blows. They are often indifferent or unaware of pain or injury to themselves. Some disorganized people target specific people to harm – combat with them is like fighting a tornado of arms and legs. Others are so "lost" that they are not fighting, per se. They are "swimming through people" – it is as if they are drowning, trying to struggle through a river, choked with wreckage, the people and objects around them the debris they are trying to force their way through. A helpful image is Taz, the whirlwind character in the old Warner Brother's cartoons.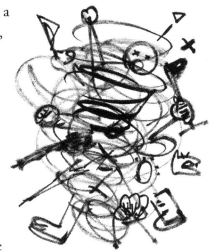

Such behaviors should be considered a medical emergency, and proper medical attention must be summoned as soon as possible – ideally, they should stage nearby while staff and/or law enforcement are establishing the safe de-escalation and resolution of the crisis. The chaotic state can be a sign of a life-threatening emergency.

It is possible that chaotic rage may be part of the behavioral profile of a severely disabled patient, one who is not necessarily in a delirium state. If such an individual is in long-term care, you must have expert consultation to ensure that staff can differentiate between an emotional storm and a medical crisis.

De-Escalation of Chaotic Rage
- Disorganized or delirious individuals are among the most difficult to verbally de-escalate, because comprehension and coherent cognitive processes are among the first faculties they lose. Because of their impulsiveness and unpredictability, you must be on guard against a sudden attack. Therefore, knowledge of anything that might have set them off in the past is very useful. This information should be highlighted in some fashion in the records of long-term patients. In crisis intervention situations, ask family members and others close to the patient if they are aware of any triggers.
- In addition to the person attempting to verbally de-escalate and control the person in the chaotic rage state, a second person needs to take command and control of the situation and direct others (clear the room of others, provide site security to prevent others from entering the area, phone for police and emergency medical assistance, coordinate physical restraint, etc.).
- Use calm movements and a firm but reassuring voice. People in chaotic states, most notably delirium, often experience poor motor control, vertigo, disorientation, etc. Slow movements and a soothing tone of voice help them orient physically and emotionally.
- Use simple, concrete commands with no more than a single "subject" in each sentence, as complex sentences or detailed instructions will be confusing, overwhelming, or irritating. Repetition is almost always helpful. For example, say slowly, "Sit down, William. Sit down. Sit down. William, sit down."

- One of the last things the disorganized person will retain is recognition of their name. Use their name repeatedly, interspersing it in your commands in order to get their attention before attempting to redirect them to another activity.
- They are susceptible to being deflected to another topic. You can sometimes simply distract the patient, although this is unlikely when they have entered fully into chaotic rage.
- You can sometimes fabricate a theme that catches their attention and seems to engage higher thought processes, delaying their outburst of rage until help can arrive.

Example: Fabrication of a theme to catch their attention

A paramedic approached a delirious man who was standing on the edge of a highway, and said, "Ike, what are you doing here? I haven't seen you since high school." As he kept rattling off fictitious memories to the man, whose name was *not* Ike and whom he had never seen before, the delirious man gazed into his eyes in confusion, rocking back and forth in rhythm with the paramedic's words. The paramedic was successful in capturing the man's attention, which kept him from dashing into traffic, until police arrived. To illustrate how dangerous this situation was, the moment the police tried to physically ease him back from the highway, the man exploded into a violent attack, requiring a number of police officers to subdue him.

- Use paraphrasing to validate and acknowledge their confusion and/or fear. For example, "Really scary, huh?" or "You are really worried, aren't you?"
- Be very cautious about touching those in chaotic rage, as this may be experienced as invasive or even as an attack.

Physical contact: guidance and restraint

Specific training is required concerning if and when to touch someone who has lost control and needs to be moved or restrained in some way. Staff should know the plan, and be ready to initiate at the signal of the lead staff person. This is NEVER a one-person operation. Staff must not only know the plan, but they must also regularly practice physical guidance and restraint procedures to keep both patients and staff safe.

If you need to touch a patient in a chaotic rage state, for example, to guide them to another room, be sure to touch them firmly. However, do not curve your fingers inward, because the tips of your fingers digging into their flesh will be interpreted as an attack. Do not stroke, pat, or caress them: although you may intend to comfort them, you have absolutely no way of knowing what emotions such touch can elicit. The proper touch is firm, in essence, telling the person, "Here is your body. Here's where it stops. This body contains you. It is that which holds you. My hand is only to inform you of your bodily existence and to show you a safe way to go."

- Do whatever you can to minimize environmental stressors. Disorganized individuals often become agitated due to light, noise, and a chaotic environment. Try to clear the room of onlookers or extraneous personnel.
- Minimize extraneous body movements and other distracting behaviors. Your movements should be calming, and also only be those useful in helping the person understand what is going on.
- Make "invasive" procedures that must be carried out as gentle and safe as possible.
- Because of their difficulty in attending to what you say, nonverbal communication is a paramount concern. A calm, reassuring presence, manifesting both strength and assurance, is truly your best hope of helping to stabilize an individual in chaotic rage.

About "Excited Delirium Syndrome": Agitated Chaos

Excited delirium is a rare condition at the extreme end of the hyper-aroused wing of the delirium spectrum. Although etiology can be varied, excited delirium is most commonly associated with long-term use of stimulants, particularly cocaine and methamphetamine, or drugs such as PCP. It is also associated with extreme manic or psychotic excitement, and can be precipitated by a variety of purely medical conditions. It is typified by some, if not all, of the following: a sudden onset of extreme agitation; pervasive terror, often without object; chaotic, sudden shifts in emotions; disorientation; communication difficulties, which may include screaming, pressured or incoherent speech, grunting, or irrational spurts of speech; aggression to inanimate objects (particularly shiny objects like glass and mirrors); hyper-arousal with unbelievable strength, endurance, and insensitivity to pain; and, most notably, hyperthermia accompanied by stripping off clothes and violent resistance to others, before, during, and after arrest or restraint.

Accompanying their almost unbelievable level of physical arousal and resistance to both physical and mechanical restraints is respiratory and cardiac arrest, appallingly high body temperature, and rhabdomyolysis (the rapid breakdown of muscle tissue that can cause renal failure), all of which can lead to death. The usual pattern is that they struggle with incredible power and then, suddenly, they stop moving. Or sometime after becoming quiet, either in a stupor or in seeming normality, they die, usually from cardiac arrest. This can look remarkably similar to a seizure, also a very dangerous syndrome.

If you are a drug treatment or detox facility, it is your responsibility to immediately call for emergency help, summoning <u>both</u> police and emergency medical teams whenever you are dealing with someone displaying some or all of these behaviors. Tell the emergency operator that the person looks like they are suffering from excited delirium and protocol demands both police and emergency medical personnel on the scene. Such individuals are appallingly dangerous both to others and to themselves. **<u>This is a medical emergency manifesting as physical danger</u>**.

If you are a psychiatric hospital or emergency room, it is very likely that patients will be brought to your unit after arrest and restraint by law enforcement. It is very likely that there was a prolonged struggle. They may have been Taser'd or received another form of electrical stimulation that causes the nervous system to react in a way that renders, for a brief period, skeletal muscles beyond one's voluntary control, thus enabling the police to safely bring the person under physical control. Very typically, the person continues to fight while in restraints. They continue to be utterly resistant to verbal de-escalation.

Please refer to the websites http://www.ipicd.com/ and http://www.exciteddelirium.org/ for vital information on "excited delirium" states. Given the increasing prevalence of this syndrome, your hospital must have a protocol for such patients, based on the latest research in this area.

You will, almost surely, be unable to verbally de-escalate such people, but if they are not presenting an immediate assault risk, make the attempt using the principles described above in regards to chaotic rage. If nothing else you will buy time, allowing sufficient emergency personnel to muster, making the restraint which will be necessary to get them help more feasible. The less time the individual struggles before they are physically controlled, be it against you, the police, or mechanical restraints, the more likely they are to survive.

Most individuals who go into chaotic rage are <u>not</u> in an excited delirium – but given the ever-increasing abuse of stimulants (methamphetamine, cocaine, etc.) that are the most common precipitants of this condition, it is important that you are familiar with the signs, symptoms, and "best-practice" interventions.

Remember! They are not safe just because they are restrained. Proper medical intervention is absolutely imperative. Otherwise, the patient may die.

Catatonia: Special Considerations

People may be immobile for many reasons. Catatonia, however, is a very rare, very bizarre condition in which a person stays in a fixed posture, not congruent with injury or seizure. Catatonia is caused either by mental illness (schizophrenia) or an organic condition (drug toxicity, for example). The catatonic person's posture may be quite awkward or twisted, seeming to require great flexibility. A classic symptom of true catatonia is "waxy immobility": if someone else moves the body or limbs, the person maintains the posture into which they were moved. Such individuals are often totally unresponsive to speech, touch, or even pain, and there seems to be no way to establish communication with them.

Considerable caution is needed in dealing with immobile individuals for several reasons. They may be injured or having a seizure and are in need of medical attention. A second consideration is safety. One way to regard catatonia is to view the patient as exerting 100 percent of their will to *not* interact with the outside world. Trying to help, you may be tempted to make physical contact or speak forcefully to them in an effort to get them to respond when they are unsecured. This can be a disastrous mistake. Imagine the incredible exertion of will required to maintain immobility for hours, even days, without movement, without response, without even blinking in some cases. Now imagine disturbing this equilibrium. The result is what is clinically called "catatonic rage," a state that can be considered one form of excited delirium. The individual shifts from 100 percent quietude to 100 percent explosive motion.

Example: The power of catatonic rage

I am aware of one incident in which a law enforcement officer's career was ended by such an individual who, all of 110 pounds, grabbed hold of his arm, and, yanking as if he was cracking a whip, ripped through all the ligaments of his shoulder and shoulder blade.

Although you may think the person is unaware, they *can* hear you. Therefore, speak calmly and respectfully. People can have very long memories of being shamed, and if you speak about or treat the catatonic as an object rather than a person, you may evoke a terrible sense of humiliation. They may not be able to respond in their "frozen" state, but months or years later, encountering another person like the one who verbally demeaned them (another nurse or doctor, for example), they may target this individual as a stand-in for their postponed rage. Beyond that, everyone, even a person in a coma, deserves to be treated with respect. Even if it seems that the person cannot hear a word that you are saying, act as if they are listening to everything you say.

With such a person, do everything in your power to ensure that staff are aware that they are dealing with someone who is very likely catatonic, and that they should not disturb them any more than is necessary. When you move them to a gurney or a bed, make sure you have sufficient numbers to safely manage them, in case they explode suddenly while being moved.

CHAPTER 58

Terrified Rage

> **The line between terrified and chaotic rage can be very fine.**
> The terrified person, overwhelmed, can shift into chaotic rage. When facing an individual in a state of either pure terror or terrified rage, be prepared, therefore, to shift to protocols suitable to assisting individuals in chaotic states (Chapter 57).

What Does Terrified Rage Look Like?

Terrified individuals believe that they will be violated or abused. They appear apprehensive and furtive, looking halfway ready to run, halfway ready to strike. Their voice can be pleading, whiny, or fearful, and their eyes are often wide open or darting from place to place. Wide-open eyes do not always indicate fear, however. When fearful, the muscles under the eyes are slack, giving their face a pleading look. Even though the terrified person is looking in your direction, they do not usually look *into* your eyes, nor do they want you to look into theirs. The enraged, aggressive individual with wide-open eyes, on the other hand, displays tension around the eyes. Furthermore, they often look penetratingly into your eyes, or *through* you.

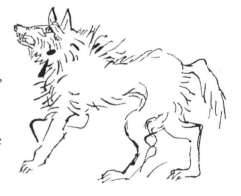

The mouth of some terrified people gapes slightly as they breathe in panicky short gasps, high in the chest, while others press their lips together in a quivering pucker. Their skin tone is often ashen or pale. Some make threatening gestures with a flailing overhand blow, while others primarily use a fending off gesture, as if trying to ward off attack. Their body posture can be described as concave, as they pull away from you, or hold themselves tightly in fear. Their body is usually tense, preparing to either defend themselves or flee. They also exhibit heightened levels of physical arousal, accompanied by panting, sweating, and trembling. They may back into a wall or corner. They may also yell, threatening and pleading at the same time, using such phrases as, "Stay back! You get away from me! I will hit you!! I will! You stay back!" There is a hollow quality to their voice, as if it has no "foundation." This is due to the tightening of their abdomen and diaphragm, so that not only their breathing, but also their speech is high in their chest.

What Causes Terrified Rage?

Severely frightened people often suffer from paranoid delusions, a fear of the unknown, or terrifying hallucinations. At other times, they are afraid of a loss of control, or of being laughed at or humiliated. Some people are afraid that they are in terrible trouble with some agency – be it police, hospital staff, or mental health professionals. Finally, for any number of reasons, they are simply terrified of you. *Imagine a snarling wolf cornered, backed up against a cliff face*.

De-Escalation of Terrified Rage

Try to reduce the terrified person's sense of danger. Maintain a safe distance and relax your posture. Make sure your movements are unhurried, and your voice is firm, confident, and reassuring.

Notice if their body relaxes or tenses in response to your eye contact or its lack. If direct eye contact is re-assuring for the person, do so; if intimidating, do not. Of course, you should never take your eyes *off* the person: the point is that you should not look penetratingly into their eyes if such contact terrifies them.

Initiate a litany of reassuring phrases, speaking slowly, with frequent pauses: "I know you are scared – that's OK. - - - - Put down the chair. - - - - You don't need that. - - - - - - - I keep it safe here. You can put it down now. - - - - - - I'm way over here. - - - - - - Go ahead. Sit down. - - - - - - - I keep it safe."

DO NOT say, "I'll protect you" or "I won't hurt you." Many people who shift into terrified rage have been hurt by people who said those kinds of phrases. However, when you say, "I keep it safe here," you are implicitly telling them, "This is my territory and no one, including you, will be hurt on my territory. I am taking responsibility now, and because of me, you will be safe." Furthermore, by saying something similar to what they expect to hear, yet somehow different, you cause a "glitch" in their thought process. "What did he say? He didn't say, 'I'll keep you safe.' What's different in what he said?'" By getting the terrified person to question what you said, you cause them to "re-engage" the parts of the brain that actually think things through as opposed to just reacting.

Their body language will also indicate that they are calming down. Their breathing will get a little shuddery or be expressed in short high-pitched gasps. They may slump into a chair or onto the floor, as if physically exhausted, or they may even begin to weep. Maintain your reassuring litany and slowly approach them. If they show signs of becoming frightened again, pause, move slightly back, and continue to speak reassuringly.

As you approach the person, move in "half steps." For example, move the right foot a full step, then bring the left foot *up* to the right foot. Pause. Move either right or left foot forward, and then bring the other foot forward *up* to the lead foot. Pause. The advantage of moving this way is that you stay balanced, in case the individual suddenly attacks. Furthermore, you can ease backward, creating more space between you if the person becomes startled or reactive.

Attempting to hold or hug the person to comfort their fears should NOT be your first choice. <u>Particularly with adults, this will be a very rare option.</u> There are some times, however, when that is the right thing to do.

With adults, touch usually occurs at the end, when they are calm, close to baseline, or even further into post-crisis depression. If touch is in order, it should be firm. Be very careful as many adults will still be frightened and confused, and can misunderstand your intentions. Therefore, <u>do not</u> try to touch them unless you have a strong sense that you will be experienced as comforting and welcome. Do not curve your hand so that the fingertips "dig" inward: your hands, particularly to the hypersensitive person, will feel like claws. You must not stroke or pat them: these are gestures that are meant to *evoke* feelings. *A firm touch is to help the person dampen down their emotions.* If you feel any tension in their body in response to your touch, calmly remove your hand. To reiterate, in such situations, touch is the <u>most rare</u> of options, but this is how to do it in cases where it is warranted. In such cases, the best touch to an adult is a firm palm of the hand on the shoulder – in particular, the deltoid muscle. If you place your hand on their trapezius muscle, you are too close to their neck. This may very likely be experienced as threatening or intrusive.

With small children, it is often very effective to wrap them very firmly in your arms, containing their rage within your kind strength. At the same time, reassure the child that you are holding them to keep them safe.

Restraining a small child, or a childlike adult

If you do wrap a child in your arms, it is often very effective to "shove" a beloved toy – such as a teddy bear or a doll – into their arms, so that they are holding the toy in the same way you are holding them. In other words, wrap the child around the toy as you wrap around them. At this time, you can repeat such phrases as, "You hold onto that dolly. Hold onto her so she won't get hurt. Hold her tight." You are subliminally suggesting that you are holding the child in the same way.

This can also be done with terrified developmentally disabled people.

When Should You Allow the Terrified Person to Leave?

Fearful people feel trapped: this is one of the primary reasons why they are frightened. Remember the image of a "cornered wolf." The last thing you should do with a wolf is to block it from escape. Aside from locked units where people must be kept from leaving, there are situations where you tell the person, "You can stay or go if you want. I am concerned for you and want to help you. But you do not have to stay if you don't want to." On the other hand, you may have a responsibility to protect both the terrified person and other people. If you are concerned that the person may run out and harm either themselves or other people, you have a professional and moral responsibility to keep them safe by keeping them close.

CHAPTER 59

Hot Rage

"Hot rage explodes when officers either can't calm them down for a variety of reasons, did not take the time to calm them down, or the officers themselves were so pissed off that they got the subject into that stage. One out of three is not our fault. Three out of three become our responsibility."

– A veteran police officer

When we think of people on the edge of violence, hot rage usually comes to mind. Imagine an individual with muscles writhing, yelling or screaming, fist brandished, threatening to harm you. They throw things, tip over desks, and spit in your face. They want to beat you bloody, stab you, or pound you into a pulp.

Such behaviors are often thought to be instinctual, a product of our primitive drives – almost a reflex. However, instinctual aggression is usually uncoordinated and flailing, and falls under the category of terrorized or chaotic rage.

Hot rage, however, is coordinated: learned through modeling, trained through repetition, and reinforced through success. This doesn't mean that hot rage is the equivalent of the actions of a professional fighter, who coolly and calmly prepares his line of attack and focuses his aggression on his opponent.

It is most productive to think of hot rage as a "pseudo instinct" – a behavior that is a combination of primitive drives and trained actions. Such pseudo-instinctual behaviors are actions that have either been repeated so often or are so ingrained through powerful early experiences that they function almost like reflexes. Hot rage also leads to deterioration in judgment, and at higher states of arousal, even basic cognitive processes. For example, some people with a history of abuse lash out in rage whenever frightened, with no ability to evaluate whether or not they are currently in danger. At the same time, they target where best to hit, and frequently choose a time and a place where they believe they have the best chance of success. On a more functional level, a good street fighter does his best to knock his opponent senseless, but he automatically takes a stance with chin tucked in, shoulder rolled forward, and punches in such a way that the power of the blow is amplified by his body weight and the torque of his hips.

General Information about Hot Rage

Hot rage is typified by emotional arousal or excitement. Arousal breeds arousal: the more often people go into hot rage states, the more comfortable they are with their rage, and the easier it becomes to be violent. There are also organic contributors: low blood sugar levels, head injury, or the use of drugs and alcohol that act as disinhibiters.

Hot rage is often a behavior that has led to short-term success in the past, such as scaring and beating a selected victim either for criminal gain or just for the joy of the beating. In a state of rage, such a person has no concern about longer-term consequences, much less guilt. Bored individuals or others who need a lot of intensity to feel alive will amp up aggression to feel this energy and power. For some people, there is a sense of liberation, even a paradoxical kind of joy, when they peak into rage. All their fears and insecurities disappear, and they merge into the ecstasy of the pure act. These individuals desire rage, because that ecstatic state is, to them, the best thing they ever feel.

Displacement is a common factor of hot rage, meaning the patient's anger is displaced, at least temporarily, toward an inanimate object instead of you or another individual. This also includes picking things up and slamming them down, throwing things, punching or kicking walls, furniture, or other nearby objects. More predatory individuals use displacement as a tactic to make the target of their aggression more fearful, while warming themselves up for an attack.

Hot rage is also associated with peer group influence and masculine display, a primitive attempt to gain status in an aggressive group, or win a perceived competition with other males in regards to objects of desire. This becomes especially problematic if the patient begins acting out in front of a group of onlookers, friends, or family; they must act aggressively toward anyone representing authority in order to save face.

Some therapeutic professionals claim that hot rage is a result of frustration, but this alone does not usually elicit rage in normal people. People are more likely to become enraged when frustrated desires are coupled with something personal, such as when the patient believes someone else is impeding them. Particularly in mental health settings, hot rage can be a transference reaction in which the staff person is a representative or stand-in for someone else. In their mind, you are the emblem of everyone who ever controlled them or put them down, an agent of an oppressive society, or simply a legitimate target for hatred and violence.

Three subtypes of hot rage, each typified by almost unendurably intense feelings, will be discussed later in this chapter. They are fury, bluffing, and aggressive-manipulation.

General De-Escalation of Hot Rage: The Ladder

The primary method of de-escalation for hot rage is called "the ladder." This is an ideal technique for someone who is beginning to get threatening. It is used only for rage, that gray zone between anger (even extreme anger) and violence. The person is presenting a danger to you, and is no longer trying to communicate with you. Instead, they are right on the edge of assault – in a sense, doing a war dance to overcome their inhibitions against committing violence.

> **The ladder should only be used with an enraged individual**
>
> Using this technique with an angry individual, even an extremely angry person will cause them to *flare up* in rage. To give a sense of proportion, despite a twenty-year career in which I have dealt with many very aggressive, profoundly dangerous people, I have only had to use the ladder twice. In every other case, de-escalation tactics suitable to dealing with angry people were sufficient.

The ladder technique itself is simple. Identify the most dangerous behavior and repetitively demand that it cease. Use a short sentence with no more than four or five words. Your tone must be strong and matter-of-fact. Once they stop that particular dangerous behavior, identify the next problematic behavior and use the same technique. Continue until the person is de-escalated. This technique is only effective right before, during, and after the peak of the crisis because it is a control tactic rather than a "lining Up" de-escalation tactic. Control tactics will provoke rage in a merely angry person, someone we might have over-estimated, due to his loud tone, or dramatic behaviors. As described above, facing an enraged person causes us to experience fear in a way that anger does not. With the enraged patient, the danger is NOW, not merely a possibility should the situation continue to deteriorate.

> **Do not:**
> - Explain yourself.
> - Use a scolding or nagging tone.
> - Request that they comply.
> - Use "psychologese," such as, "It's not appropriate for you to . . ."

Establish a Hierarchy of Danger

The general hierarchy from most to least is as follows:

1. Brandishing an object or a weapon in a menacing way. (**NOTE**: If they are too close or are trying to use the weapon, this is **violence**, not rage. In this case, try to establish safety, not control.)
2. Approaching or standing too close to you with menacing intent.
3. Kicking objects, punching walls, or throwing things (displacement activity).
4. Pacing, stomping, and inflating the body in an aggressive manner (posturing).
5. Shouting *or* talking in low, menacing tones.
6. Using language that is intended to violate, demean or degrade.

The ladder is not merely a verbal intervention. Like any other control tactic with an aggressive patient, you must move as needed to maintain the optimum space to both defend yourself and exert maximum influence upon the aggressor. If they are very close, or threatening, your hands should be up, palms out, fingertips curved, prepared to ward off any attack, but also as a gesture that is both calming and dominant.

Give the aggressor a straightforward command to stop their most dangerous behavior. You should not scream or shout – that will not get through to the person. Instead, they will ramp up on your screaming tone, and this alone will increase their aggressive energy. Rather, your voice should be strong, low, and commanding (Chapter 39).

After every couple of repetitions, always add, "We'll talk about it when you . . ." followed by the same command. Once that behavior is stopped, pick the next most problematic behavior (the next "rung" of the ladder), and command/require that it stop. If the person does calm down and stops <u>all</u> the aggressive behaviors, including assaultive language, THEN set a firm and direct limit.

This is not the time to try to think of something brilliant or life changing to say. By keeping things simple, you can continue to look for escape routes, identify potential weapons, and attempt to get help. Intersperse their name frequently in your sentences, using this to pace and break the rhythm of your commands and to "call them back" to a more personal interaction. In addition, by holding to a demand that a specific behavior cease you are displaying clarity and strength to the patient, as well as helping him focus *their* mind on their most problematic behavior, then the next, and on down the rungs of the ladder.

Continue working your way down the rungs until the patient is no longer in a state of fury. If the patient re-escalates to a higher and more dangerous activity, simply return to that rung of the ladder and begin again. Remember to stand and use your voice as described in the previous sections.

The last "rung" is probably swearing or other obscene language. Remember, people swear as "punctuation," without hostile intent. They may be crude, but they are not trying to be verbally violent. If the person is swearing in this manner, it is not a problem. That is something you will deal with at another time, during moments of calm, saying, for example, "Jamey, I don't like to hear that kind of language. I'd appreciate if you don't swear around me."

However, if the swearing is an attempt to violate you, it <u>must</u> be dealt with in proper order. However, do <u>not</u> focus on the language, no matter how vile, if the person is *doing* something dangerous. Remember that predatory individuals will use language to shock, distract, immobilize or terrorize. What they are <u>doing</u> is far more dangerous than what they are saying.

Safety above all

If your client becomes violent, do not hold back from any action to keep yourself and others safe. If you do have to protect yourself and/or others, do so! Escape, evade, restrain, and even fight back, if that is what you have to do. Verbal control tactics are, of course, ideal with people in a state of rage, but if they cross the line into violence, do what you have to do to stay safe.

Example: The ladder technique

Your voice is firm, low-pitched, and commanding as you "descend" the rungs. Each statement is, of course, in response to something the aggressor has done or said. Do not talk too fast. (Note the <pause> notation within the first couple of phrases below. You do this with every statement. The pauses should be of different lengths, breaking the rhythm, rather than counting cadence.)

"Step back. <pause> Step back. Robert. <pause> We'll talk about it when you step back. <pause> Robert. <pause> Step back. Step back, Robert. <pause> We will talk about it when you step back."

"Stop kicking things. Robert. Stop kicking things. We'll talk about it when you stop kicking things."

"Robert, I cannot follow you when you pace around. Sit down and we'll talk. Sit down, Robert."

Notice the paradoxical message that you cannot "follow" them. Aside from this having a double meaning ("follow" also means to understand), of course you can follow them. You are also trying to catch their attention as they try to figure out the sense of what you said. This draws in the higher areas of the brain – the neo-cortex –that actually tries to think through a problem. Once reactivated, the person is less likely to be assaultive. (This was referred to as a "brain glitch" in Chapter 57.)

Imagine they have stepped forward again, thus ascending to a higher "rung" on the ladder.

"Step back! Robert! Step back and we'll talk. We will TALK about it when you step back, Robert. Step - - - - - back."

"Sit down, Robert. We will talk about it when you sit down. We cannot talk when you are walking around. We will talk about it when you sit down."

"Lower your voice. I cannot hear you when you yell that loud. Lower you voice and we will talk."

Here is a second paradoxical communication – of course, you can hear a person who is shouting. Once again, you are trying to create a "glitch" where the aggressive person tries to figure out what you mean when you say you cannot hear him when he is yelling.

"Talk to me with the same respect that I talk to you. We will talk about it when you stop swearing. Stop swearing. Robert. Talk to me with respect, the same way I talk to you."

You continue to work your way down the "rungs" until the person is no longer in a state of fury. As you see, if the person re-escalates to a higher and more dangerous activity, simply go up to that "rung" of the ladder and begin repeating that command again. Remember to stand and use your voice as described in the previous sections. Usually, the last rung is shouting, or even further down – swearing and using demeaning, ugly language.

Limit Setting after De-Escalation

Once the person is stable and willing to talk, it is important to clearly set a limit.

Remember, you have not merely de-escalated an angry individual – you have *controlled* someone on the edge of violence, someone who almost assaulted you or another person. You must not relinquish that control now. Depending on the circumstances, here is what will happen next:

- Particularly when there has been property destruction or near assault, the person should be escorted off the premises by police, security, or staff, or even immediately arrested. The aggressor can be given a trespass warning by police, forbidding them to return to your hospital. You may also discuss other charges with the police, such as assault, destruction of property, threatening a health care worker, or disruption of a health care facility.

- Sometimes you will require the person to leave your office or agency even without police or security response.

- In some inpatient units, the enraged person will either be escorted to or restrained and conveyed to a seclusion room for a period of time.

- You will sometimes set up a meeting for later. When this will be depends on the type of milieu. With non-hospitalized individuals, such as family members, you may set up a phone call to *discuss* setting up a meeting.

- With cognitively impaired individuals, you may merely request that they sit quietly and continue to calm themselves, that you will meet with them in ten or twenty minutes. It is usually NOT a good idea to process or discuss the recent incident. It is very likely that they will feel "existentially wrong" – that you are attacking them. Education on better ways to handle upset should take place at another time, when they are totally calm.

Example: Limit setting

As each person and situation is different, you will have to adapt as needed. In this example, the patient has mostly postured, but they also brandished a fist. They did not become so aggressive that they needed to be physically restrained.

"Robert, you have physically threatened me and used obscene language toward me. I will not accept anyone trying to intimidate or abuse me. I would like us to take a break from each other. You can go to your room or you can go to the lounge. I'm going back to my office now. We can talk about your court hearing later. But not right now. "

(Imagine the person objects at this point and says, "You said we would talk about it!) You should reply, "We are talking about *it*! What we are talking about is that you threatened violence. We cannot get anything accomplished if you are going to do that. I know you were very upset. You know that we never solve any problem when that happens. Let's talk about it again when both of us are feeling peaceful. I have some free time at 2 p.m. today. I'll be happy to see you then. But when you return, I expect you to treat me with the same respect I treat you, without threats, and without cursing or yelling. We can and will talk about your concerns. But that will be later, when we can easily talk about it. Not now. "

Hot Rage Subtype #1: Fury

What does fury look like? Furious people are very tense, looking as if they are about to explode. If they are large in stature, imagine a grizzly bear; if they are smaller, imagine a wolverine. In either case, the image suggests a being that will tear you to pieces if it perceives danger, is provoked, or is cornered. Many people, both with mental health diagnoses and without, display fury, and it is particularly common among people who have suffered head injuries. Furious patients may show some of the following physical manifestations of their rage:

- Their skin tone is flushed as they become angered, turning red or purplish. As they become even more enraged, however, their skin blanches, and they turn pale or gray (depending on their skin color), as the blood pools in the internal organs.
- Their voice, whether loud or low and quiet, has a menacing and belligerent tone.
- They often pace, inflate their upper body, hit or kick objects, or strike their hands together ominously, punching one fist into the other hand.
- They tend to stare into your eyes directly, glowering from under their brow, with a furious and hostile look on their face.
- Their eyes will appear red or inflamed; usually their eyes are wide open, with tension around the eye sockets and facial muscles.
- Physical arousal, blood pressure, and muscular tension all increase. You may notice veins popping out of the skin, particularly around the neck.
- They may display a smile that shows no humor or joy. Others snarl or compress their lips with a twist, as if they have a foul taste in their mouth. Still others bare their teeth or clench their jaws so tightly that the muscles stand out in bunches.

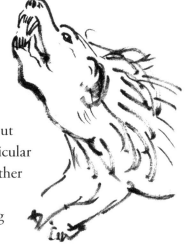

- They are very impulsive and unconcerned with possible consequences.
- Their breathing is often loud and straining.
- They may claim to be disrespected, humiliated, or shamed. Others will allege that they are not getting their questions answered and their problem solved, or that no one is listening or cares. They may rant about "the system" and claim that they are out of alternatives or solutions. (These verbalizations are for a particular audience – themselves – functioning as a feedback loop to further escalate themselves.)
- At their most dangerous point, they may become calm, breaking off eye contact, or adopt a thousand-yard stare.

Control of Fury

When confronting a furious individual, your posture and tone should be confident, commanding, even imposing. Maintain direct eye contact and frequently use their name.

Stand directly in front of the individual, but out of range of an immediate blow. Stand too close and you will appear to be challenging the patient, too far and you will be seen as fearful, a potential victim. You may have to move forward or backward to maintain this spacing. In either event, move smoothly, flinching on the one hand or any sudden or threatening gestures on the other. When you move with a relaxed body, you are more ready to protect yourself, yet you do not appear as if you are trying to initiate a physical altercation.

Do not square your feet so that you are confronting him in full frontal fashion; stand with your feet in a "blade" stance, with one foot advanced, and the other behind at about a 45-degree angle. (If you drew the back foot forward, there would be one or two fist's space between the heels – do not line the feet up, one behind the other.) This prepares you to escape along tangents to his attack, to ward off blows, and if necessary, to fight back. With the blade stance, you are already "chambered" to do this. As described earlier, your hands are either up in a fence, or the wrist of one arm is clasped in the hand of the other in front of you at waist level (Chapter 38).

Your voice is strong and forceful. Do not, however, shout. Instead, keep your voice low-pitched and calm, dropping it into your chest where it resonates, as enraged people, in particular, react violently to threatening or angry vocal tones. The only time you would shout is a "battle cry," that lion's roar of outrage and strength that you use only when you are trying to stop an actual attack.

You will use the ladder in its most orthodox form – with your voice pitched low and powerful. You should feel it vibrate in your chest.

The individual will exhibit one of three actions:

- They keep on coming. You will do what you have to do to ensure safety.
- They get close and when you tell them to step back, they say, "Make me." You will do what you have to do to ensure safety.
- They comply. When individuals in hot rage comply with the command to step back, they usually do so yelling and screaming, "You can't tell me what to do."

Once you have them de-escalated, you must maintain control. As previously stated in the section on limit setting, only after setting very strong limits will you shift into problem solving, even with a mentally ill individual. Otherwise, they will assume that the best way to get a reward – your attention or help – is to abuse you.

Hot Rage Subtype #2: Enraged Bluffing

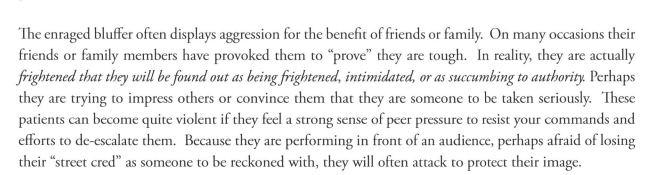

In keeping with the "animal behavior" analogy when describing the furious patient, the aggressively bluffing patient is like a gorilla beating his chest, a display of aggression designed to keep you at a distance. There is a sense of bluster rather than the pent-up pressure of the enraged person. They are like a wind blowing against a stone wall rather than pent-up explosiveness of dynamite under a rock. However, their manifest behavior appears much the same as the individual displaying fury, hence the terrifying image of the enraged gorilla. At 50 yards, could you tell the difference between a charging gorilla and a charging grizzly bear? Both are huge, hairy beasts that apparently mean you harm. In all likelihood, the gorilla would prefer to be left alone rather than engage in combat, but he postures as if he wants nothing more than to tear you to pieces. If he perceives no other alternative, he will do so.

The enraged bluffer often displays aggression for the benefit of friends or family. On many occasions their friends or family members have provoked them to "prove" they are tough. In reality, they are actually *frightened that they will be found out as being frightened, intimidated, or as succumbing to authority.* Perhaps they are trying to impress others or convince them that they are someone to be taken seriously. These patients can become quite violent if they feel a strong sense of peer pressure to resist your commands and efforts to de-escalate them. Because they are performing in front of an audience, perhaps afraid of losing their "street cred" as someone to be reckoned with, they will often attack to protect their image.

Sometimes bluffers are alone, but they still have an audience, one inside their own head. They have an image in their mind, and they believe they must conform to that image. You will often hear this in their self-talk as they amp themselves up: "You don't know who you are talking to. Do you believe this guy? Do you have any idea who I am?"

Many bullies who have a long record of violence actually function in bluff mode. They are in a perpetual quest to prove to others, and even more insidiously, to themselves, that they are not frightened. As a result, they repetitively solicit situations where they must either intimidate or beat someone bloody. It is essential, therefore, to short circuit this behavior before it escalates into violence. Obviously, one of the most important steps toward achieving this is to separate the enraged bluffer from his or her audience. At the same time, you should not, thereby, isolate yourself with the enraged person without sufficient backup.

How can you tell the difference between a person in hot fury as opposed to a bluffer if their behaviors are so much the same? When we are facing a furious person, fear is a natural and likely response. Your instinctual mind, that part of you that puts survival above all else, demands your immediate attention, and it uses fear to accomplish this. An aggressive bluffer, in a state of hot rage, may also elicit fear, but this fear will be accompanied by another emotion: you will find yourself a bit irritated, thinking how stupid (yet potentially dangerous) this incident has become, and that if the bluffer was not with his friends, or in another case, if his wife had not chosen to taunt him as being less than a man, this dangerous situation would never have developed.

One thing that you simply cannot do is to try and "out tough" the bluffer by refusing to back down or leave the scene. This is merely bluffing behavior on your part, and the aggressor's audience will only amplify their calls for them to be even more resistant. Do not personalize encounters with your patients, and if professional prudence dictates that you should retreat, then do so!

Control of Bluffing

These individuals are not really in confrontation with you. They are *pretending* that they are. But this is a pretense that can kill. This pretense is usually for an audience, but sometimes they are trying to *stand up the image they wish to project to the world.* These patients remain quite dangerous because they may believe they need to prove themselves by refusing to back down. Another aspect of bluffing is that when frightened, the bluffing patient will move forward, toward you, so that no one will see how frightened they truly are.

De-escalate and control using the ladder much as you would with an individual in fury, but with a much more matter-of-fact tone. Your eye contact, too, is matter-of-fact, as if you are having a conversation rather than a confrontation. Rather than having your hands in front of you (clasped or in a fence position), open your hands, slightly to the sides, palms up. You can still protect yourself, but your posture appears nonthreatening, more open and relaxed. Your body language says, "There is no need for a fight here." Remember, enraged bluffers will attack out of the fear of being "found out" by their peers. Your task becomes helping them to save face, rather than issuing forceful commands and instructions. In doing so, you will greatly reduce the risk of violence.

In some situations, they are working themselves up in front of their audience, and you can short circuit things by helping them save face. Include in your strategy some information and reassurance. For example, you can say, "Look, Frank. I know you thought I was making fun of you, but that wasn't the case at all. I was just pointing out that you forgot your meds, so you wouldn't have to come back for them later." However, if they have ramped themselves into true "bluff rage," they may view concession or agreement as backing down, and only by taking control will you be able to ensure your own and other's safety.

When exerting verbal control upon the enraged bluffer, remember the following:
- Do not point out their fears in front of others. They will feel the need to defend their honor.
- Do not try to be more forceful than they are, or appear overly domineering or condescending, as their self-image may require them to strike out.
- In some situations, let them have the last word. By letting them feel a semblance of control (the half step of space that you give them), their need to appear to others as unafraid can be satisfied. When such people are given a face-saving way out, they don't feel the need to bluff or aggress further.

The bluffer's strut

When you have done things well, aggressive bluffers often strut back with a smirk, sometimes glancing around and making eye contact with onlookers. This is for the benefit of the audience, and for their own self-image. They are trying to show that they are not afraid, and in control of the situation.

- If they are not responsive to your more low-key approach and continue to escalate, you may have a furious person who happens to be in front of other people or a bluffer who has *shifted* into fury. In this case, you "turn up the dial," adopting a more powerful tone and stance, and shift into the more forceful version of the ladder technique for the furious individual. In essence, you would say, "Move back, Stephen. We will talk about it - - - - MOVE BACK." You shift from a calm ease to a powerful, adamant stance.
- Remember, it is the audience that makes them so dangerous. If possible, separating them from their audience will often result in their calming down on their own. Whenever possible, do not allow a confrontation to take place in front of a person's retinue of friends and family.

Setting Consequences with a Person Who Has Enacted Enraged Bluff

Just as with the furious person, you must set limits at the end of the confrontation. However, you should also include some "ego building." These individuals are most dangerous when they believe they must create a fearsome or frightening impression on other people. Therefore, draw them aside and say something like, "Bernard, I'm glad this worked out with no one getting hurt. Had you not chosen to sit down and talk, you very likely would have ended up being taken out of here. Staff was just about to call police. No. Listen to me for a minute. I'm not disrespecting you – that's <u>why</u> you and I are over here talking instead of in front of them *<indicating the onlookers>*. Police haven't been called, but I'm telling you, it was a very near thing. Again, I'm glad this has worked out that you and I are standing here talking.

Next time, though, don't do this in front of them." ("Them" refers to his friends or family for whom he was on display. Actually, put a little *contempt* in your voice when you say the word "them," as if to indicate that Bernard is better/cooler/stronger than those people he is, in fact, trying to impress.) "Come and talk to me one man to another." (Or "one woman to another" or "one adult to another" in male-female conversations.) "You shouldn't put your personal business in front of them." You will see him visibly "puff up," feeling flattered. You then continue, "OK. Are we clear for next time? Good. Now as for this time . . ." Then, set the same types of limits as you did with the person in a state of fury.

Remember, it is the audience that makes this person most dangerous. If he feels that he will get his "respect" by himself, if he believes his status will actually improve if he comes in alone rather than with his crew of friends or family, he will be far less dangerous next time.

Hot Rage Subtype #3: Controlling, Aggressive Manipulation

What does aggressive manipulation look like?

Aggressive manipulation is a *strategy*, not a symptom of illness. Such people are calculating, trying to monitor the effect of what they are doing. They are not constrained by feelings of honor, integrity, or pride; their goal is win any way they can. You can sometimes tell when you are being manipulated ("played") because you are confused about why the person is upset or the purpose of his argument. The aggressive manipulator frequently changes either his mood or the subject of the complaint, displaying some or all of the behaviors of manipulative and psychopathic individuals (Chapters 12 and 13).

The image of a large rat is very useful when discussing the aggressive manipulator, because rats are the ultimate survivors. They will do whatever it takes to win. This image is not intended to be demeaning. It merely underscores that aggressive manipulators, like our furry, long-tailed cousins, are infinitely adaptable, and whatever the conditions, will attempt to find a way to endure or win.

Aggressive-manipulative people may have a long history of losing control, particularly when their desires are frustrated, or when they believe they are not given that which they believe they are entitled. These individuals may approach you with flattery, or a plea for something, with detailed laments about their suffering. Once their request is denied, however, they blame or criticize you for their troubles, inferring that your refusal will result in furthering their suffering or cause them irreparable harm. They might try to make you feel guilty, or begin to demean you, then shift into threats of violence. They may talk in an arrogant manner, trying to make you look incompetent to others, or stupid to yourself. They often claim to be a victim, based on either real or imagined issues. Furthermore, they may use their "status" as a member of an oppressed or victimized class of people as a means of intimidating others, making their demands in a whiny, accusatory voice. They will footnote old grievances, bringing up trivia, accusations, and old history. They will tell you how you are just like someone else who did them wrong. They will ask frequent or repetitive questions. They will try to frighten you or make you feel uncertain of yourself.

Manipulation does not mean false threat. Manipulative people will often harm others: some will even kill. The difference between such an aggressive-manipulator and those in a state of pure fury is that the furious person's inhibitions are swept aside by their rage. You will often hear terms like "he just lost it" to explain such behavior. The aggressive manipulator, on the other hand, attempts to monitor your responses and the situation as a whole to assess if their actions and behaviors are successful. Although the patient's behavior may be calculating, that does not mean they are in control. As they becomes more and more agitated, their judgment deteriorates, and they may concoct a rationalization for violence that makes sense to them in the moment, even if it would to no one else. The idea of "intimidation for next time" is the driver of some aggressive manipulator's behavior.

Examples: The aggressive-manipulative person's rationalizations
- "They say I'm mentally ill. So, just like last time, they'll plead it down to a misdemeanor and I won't really get in that much trouble."
- "If I hit her, the people here will be scared of me, and next time, they'll do what I want."
- "If I make staff here scared of me, they'll try to avoid me, and I'll have more freedom to get close to that woman who sits alone on the bench in the day room. She looks so lonely that if I act kind and sympathetic, she'll stay quiet. And with staff avoiding me, I'll have all the time I need."

Control Tactics for Aggressive Manipulators

If you recognize manipulative aggression early in your interaction with the person, you can often cut it off at the onset. For example, in a firm tone say, "Shauna, let's not even get started with this. No. I have nothing to do with medication policy here; therefore, not only will I not talk to the psychiatrist about your meds, but also you and I should not speak about it. If you are concerned, speak with your case manager. I am the wrong person to talk about this, and I don't want to waste either your time or mine." If, however, the manipulative person begins to escalate his or her strategies, you may have to use the ladder, as a means of control and de-escalation. In this case, however, your tone of voice should be matter-of-fact and slightly detached.

Making eye contact enables another person to truly see you as you are, and in return, see them as well. Aggressive-manipulative people do not care about you, and they use apparent feelings of contact and intimacy to "read" and control you. They are interested in gaining information that they can use to their benefit. Similarly, they will use their own eyes to create a (false) sense of trust to confuse you, misdirect your attention, or dominate you.

Rather than making eye contact with such people, look past one ear. Do not look away, however. While looking past an ear, you can still see what they are doing. If you look away, you will be assaulted before you even know what is coming. Your disengaged look indicates that you will not collude with them or participate in their manipulative behaviors.

The Ladder for Aggressive Manipulators

If your attempts at control and de-escalation of their manipulative strategies are unsuccessful, they may ramp up into a rage state. What distinguishes this from pure fury is that, even now, they continue to try to read and monitor you for advantage: Are they intimidating you? Have they succeeded in distracting or throwing you off balance so that you are open to an attack? Have they got you trying to "bargain" your way to safety? At the same time, they begin to "lose it," as it becomes more apparent that their strategic application of intimidation is unsuccessful. Furthermore, they get increasingly frustrated because they believe their manipulation *should* be working, primarily because it has worked so well in the past.

- Stand relaxed and ready to evade a blow and counter the attack.
- Express flat disinterest in their demands, accusations, and complaints.
- Use the repetitive commands of the ladder technique. Your vocal tone should be flat. Do not negotiate. Do not discuss other matters as long as the manipulative behavior continues.

Locking eyes: the loop

If the manipulative patient escalates into *fury*, or if they continue to be otherwise non-compliant, shift from looking past their ear to looking right in their eyes, accompanied by a firm command to stop what they are doing. <u>When you turn your head, roll it slightly up and then down as if sighting a weapon in a loop.</u> Speak powerfully and directly, just as you do with the patient who is in a state of fury. If you have ever raised a teenager, you have almost surely done this. In essence, once you make eye contact with the aggressive-manipulative patient, treat them as you would the furious type.

With the aggressive-manipulative individual, several things can happen when you attempt to control their escalation:

- Your flat disinterest means to them that they cannot "get to you." After trying several different avenues, they give up: leaving in frustration, shifting to another strategy, or sagging in defeat.
- In more heated situations, they will flare into a fury (or pseudo-fury).
- When you "loop into" eye contact, they may "bounce" off into another tactic – sudden tears, for example.
- If they do not stop immediately upon being "hit" with your eyes, this means that an attack is likely. You will shift into the de-escalation for fury or even further; take action to ensure your safety in the event of violence.

CHAPTER 60

Predatory or Cool Rage

This type of person is, thankfully, rather rare. They are intimidators who threaten either with vague innuendoes or explicit threats. Their aggressive behavior is calculated, but unlike the manipulator, violence is often their first choice rather than one of many options. The predator delivers threats in cool, dangerous tones, often *after* a clear and strongly stated demand. Then they offer you a chance to avoid injury if you comply. A variant tactic is to pretend to be out of control. (This is in contrast to a genuine attack, an action that they are eminently capable of and willing to carry out.) <u>A symbol for them is either a leopard or a shark, depending on if they present as "warm-blooded" or "stone cold."</u>

While predatory individuals seethe with hostility and/or contempt for other people, they have developed these emotions as a deliberate weapon of terror, perhaps even enjoyment. Paradoxically, their physical arousal is often low. Their heart rate can actually go down as they become more aggressive, and they can be charming and engaging, even as they are preparing to commit an act of violence. This disconnect between appearances and intentions can cause you to lower your guard because you may have a hard time believing that they are so willing to psychologically terrorize or physically hurt others, as they seem to be such nice people.

Predatory individuals actually have no inhibitions about their aggression other than tactical calculation or self-interest. They have no capacity for sympathy or guilt, and many experience low levels of anxiety in situations that would frighten ordinary people. Every time they intimidate someone successfully, their behavior is reinforced, and they view non-action on your part, either during the confrontation or afterward, as either weakness or tacit approval of their behavior, thereby increasing the likelihood of similar behavior in the future.

Your Response to the Predator

Demonstrate that you are not prey, that you are not a ready victim, and that their attempts at intimidation will not work. Most predatory individuals do not wish to interact with someone whom they *do not* intimidate or otherwise control through emotional abuse or physical posturing. Instead, they seek more conciliatory and subservient victims, where their chances of success are great. If you demonstrate that you are not prey, why don't they want to attack? It may be that they see you as another predator, one with whom he or she does not want to compete. That is not necessary, however. It is enough that he simply sees you as not "edible," like an animal with quills or one that would taste bad.

Stand or sit ready to move. Be poised, but do not appear fearful or too defensive.

Avoid gesturing or expressive movements. Fear often causes your movements to be awkward, and a predatory individual will see this as confirmation of their control over you.

Be open and strategic in everything you do: the way you position your body, your voice, and your posture. The predatory individual is well versed in reading body language and assessing weakness. Protect yourself openly, and do not change your actions based on what they say (for example they may try to put you at ease or promise compliance). The predator may use anything you do against you, either deriding you or pretending that you are out of control, paranoid, or acting strangely. Ignore all that, and openly act to keep yourself safe.

Do not overreact to vague threats, or he will interpret your reaction as a victory. An explicit threat is a criminal act. Contact law enforcement for help as soon as you can.

Cryptic Consequences

Keep your voice matter-of-fact, and give clear and direct statements of *potential* consequences. If you can, slightly smile. These consequences are of a special type – clear, but cryptic: "You know what would happen if you did hit me." In this case, do not tell them what would happen. Let their imagination take over. These vague consequences are a mirror of their own method of intimidation, and they may likely react to you as "not prey, not edible, not worth the trouble." Do not make explicit or unrealistic threats such as, "If you come near my family, I will kill you!" To the predator, that tells him what you will not do. In his mind, if you really meant it, you would do it now. An explicit threat is an empty threat.

- If they say, "What are you talking about?" you should reply, "You know exactly what we are talking about." When the predator responds to your cryptic consequence with questions or with confusing statements that would make your statement illogical, simply say, "You know what is going on here. You know what is happening."
- You may have to intersperse your vague consequences with ladder commands if they escalate their behaviors.
- Try to minimize eye contact. However, you need to look directly at them, so look between their eyes, or look at them with a flat stare. (Imagine turning your eyes to buttons. They will begin to look like a cut-out or silhouette.) Your eyes are flat, with no attempt to "penetrate" or make contact.
- You should make sustained eye contact only if in a fight for your life. Then, you must shift focus, trying to penetrate their eyes as if you were a laser beam.
- Do not overreact to their threats, or they will interpret your reaction as a victory.

The most rare of tactics

ONLY use the strategy of cryptic consequences with the openly predatory, that most rare of people, ONLY when they are escalating into predatory rage, <u>and ONLY when you have no way of escaping and summoning help</u>. In other words, it is very unlikely that these circumstances will happen, but you need to know what to do if they do.

Your entire goal is to convince them that it is not worth it to hurt you. Once you have succeeded and are free, you need to get help – almost surely from the police. To reiterate, you do not have to prove that you are bigger, tougher, or more dangerous. You are merely establishing that you are on to their game, and are not, by nature, someone to victimize. Like a leopard that chooses *not* to chase an antelope because it is moving too smoothly, obviously showing that it is healthy and strong, the predator will likely to disengage if you do not act like vulnerable prey. Therefore, do not give them anything to discount (an attempt to directly intimidate him with a direct threat) and do not try to find middle ground (negotiation is something they have no interest in – all negotiation means is that "you have given me half of what I want, let's discuss how you will give me the other half").

If, at any time, you can separate yourself from the predator, do so! Similarly, if you use these cryptic consequences and, as is very likely, they leave, dissuaded that you are not easy prey, get help! Do not keep the incident to yourself. You and your family are being threatened, whether the tone is velvet or harsh. Talk to your supervisor and hospital security, and more important, <u>speak with the police</u>. You will need advice on how to be on your guard and how best to keep everyone safe. Such incidents are sometimes a one-time affair, but on other occasions, they can go on for a long time, with further threats, stalking, or other dangerous behaviors that require you to have professional assistance to ensure that you and your family are protected.

Example: Interaction with a predatory individual when there is no escape or immediate help

Predator: "Look, this is very simple. I think you and I can agree that you misinterpreted what I said about punishing my child. I don't know where you got the idea that I said I beat her. Hey, I understand. You must have been having a bad day, and you over-reacted. This can be fixed very easily. Just call Child Protective Services and tell them that you didn't quote me accurately, that you've been overworked lately and misjudged the situation. See, I bet you love your family as much as I do. You've got your child in a good school over at Echo Lake. Actually, it's amazing, that's one of the last schools in this area that still lets the kids out for recess . . . Oh, sorry, I'm a little off track. What I'm saying is that I bet you would be devastated if anything happened to your family. I'm the same. The problem is that what is happening to my family is you! And this is a problem you could fix, unless you are really sitting there telling me that you *want* to destroy my life and that of my child. IS THAT WHAT YOU ARE SAYING! *<In silken tones>* Oh, sorry for yelling. It's just that this situation you put my family in has upset me so much."

You *(with a little smile and a strong, confident voice)*: "I am really glad we are having this conversation, because it's *good* that we both understand each other."

Predator: "So you'll make the call."

You: "Oh, I didn't say that. You know what's going to happen."

Predator: "Suppose you tell me."

You: "There's no need to do that. You know exactly what's going on."

Predator: "Are you threatening me?"

You: "I don't know where you got that idea. In fact, we both know the situation here."

Predator *(walking out)*: "You think this is over? You better watch your back."

CHAPTER 61

De-escalation of Developmentally
Disabled Individuals:
Special Considerations

Developmentally disabled people can present special challenges when they are aggressive. Many of the standard de-escalation tactics described in the chapters above are eminently useful, but you must be aware of their limitations. Keep your communications simple and direct. If you use language that is too sophisticated, either in terms of meaning or nuance, you may elicit more frustration and anger within the person by making them "feel stupid." In addition, many developmentally disabled people are subject to "magical thinking" (Chapter 14), and their beliefs about the world and their own powers and vulnerabilities often don't conform to reality. You can sometimes use these beliefs to help calm them, as you would with a child. On other occasions, you must be aware of these beliefs to keep the situation from escalating out of control.

If you try to control an agitated developmentally disabled individual based on their physical age and appearance, say a 250-pound, 35-year-old male, for example, things usually go very wrong, very quickly.

Once we make eye contact, we can usually estimate the emotional age of the developmentally disabled person: small child, young kid, preteen, or teen. **In ordinary conversation, speak to them as one does any child, drawing them "up" toward maturity: in a crisis, speak to them at their emotional age level**. However, regardless of the person's emotional age, you cannot allow their apparent childishness to compromise your physical safety. As with children, developmentally delayed people can be quite impulsive and unpredictable. Unlike children, however, they have the physical strength of an adult, and, even more dangerous, they often do not recognize their own strength. For this reason, always be ready to evade an attack and protect yourself if necessary.

Example: Speaking to the emotional age
A developmentally disabled woman grabbed my finger, trying to break it. I neutralized her attempt by shifting the angle of my hand as she yanked. Because she was at the emotional age of an eight year old, rather than forcefully commanding her to "let go!" I said, "I know you want to hold my hand. You don't have to twist my finger. We can hold hands as much as you like. Sure, we can hold hands. " She suddenly let go and dropped to the floor crying.

You can still use paraphrasing (Chapter 43) with an enraged developmentally disabled person. In this case, however, do not just calmly sum things up. Use an almost dramatic voice, over-emphasizing words. For example, you can say, "YOU are REALLLLLY mad. You are SO upset about dinner." Your voice is a combination of drama and enthusiasm. In essence, you are trying to catch their attention with charisma, a kind of energy in which you change the dynamics of your relationship through your voice and demeanor. Your dramatic voice validates how important the situation is to the angry or enraged individual.

You can use this same communication style with a developmentally disabled person who is disappointed or unhappy. "Wow. You REALLY loved that puppy! I KNOW that. You really wanted to take care of him!" Your dramatic voice validates how important the situation is to the other person – and it is the voice, here, more than the words, that provides the validation.

Talking with the Developmentally Disabled Patient after a Crisis

It is certainly reasonable to validate feelings, both for yourself and for your patient, after a crisis. For example, you might say, "Franny, that was really scary. I was scared too. I'm glad that's over. I'd like you to go to your room and have a rest. No, you are not in trouble."

A detailed critique or discussion, however, is a mistake. The cognitive limitations of developmentally disabled people affects their memory, particularly in regards to emotionally charged events. Their feelings, also, are not under their control, and they very likely will react to your debriefing as if it is a new attack, especially as you may be somewhat upset yourself by the recent incident. Your concern should be behavioral stability (no new attack) and reassurance (because they are likely afraid that you want to get back at them).

You may impose consequences in some situations. It's very important that you do not make it a punishment. Your attitude should not be, "I'll show you! You won't try that again!" Instead, consequences are a kind of reminder, something that they bump up against, in the same way that a closed door reminds one simply to not walk through it. Unless they have done something entirely new and unexpected, they should already have been told what the consequence will be if they do a particular unwanted or forbidden behavior. Consequences should be predictable, consistent, and not for the purpose of breaking their will or hurting their feelings.

CHAPTER 62

When Facing Violence

Establish Safety: What to Do If an Enraged Person Becomes Violent

Safety is defined by what you must protect. This includes yourself, other vulnerable people, and, of course, the patient, as best you can within the circumstances you are facing.

When confronted by an individual who is much more powerful, who may be armed, or who is on display in front of his confederates who may also attack, a "tactical" retreat is the best thing to do. You take the target of that person's rage, *you*, out of the picture.

Tactical retreat strategy is important with people across the range of aggression, whenever it is clear that the situation is only going to get worse and there really is nothing you can do to make it better. Whenever you can, the best thing to do is to escape and get help.

The Right to Defend Yourself: A Passage from Earlier in the Text Worth Repeating

If you are responsible for the protection of others, such as small children, or if you are trapped, you may have to fight back. In the event of an actual assault when escape is impossible, it is an absolute human right to fight to protect yourself and other potential victims. That the aggressor may also be a suffering individual does not abrogate this right. I, like you, hope that you will never face such a horrible situation. At the same time, it is necessary to be clear with yourself, on a mental and spiritual basis, that you are willing to act in defense of yourself and others. You must do this now. Trying to discover this within yourself once the assault is occurring is far too late. Remember that protecting yourself is not only a personal matter. You are protecting everyone who cares for you from the harm that they will suffer if you are maimed or killed.

Self-defense tactics are well beyond the scope of this book. Those interested should consult with recognized experts in the field to find a self-defense program suitable for your needs. The essential principle of self-defense, however, is simple:

Imagine a door with seven locks and no keys. You are locked behind the door, and all that is good in life – your family, your love, your dreams, your values, even your integrity and dignity – is secured on the other side of the door. How will you go through the door? The answer, of course, is any way you can – with tooth and nail, and any implement you can reach. A violent aggressor is that "door." You have a perfect right to be on the other side.[33]

CHAPTER 63

A Show-of-support

A show-of-support (which is sometimes called a show-of-force) is a mark of solidarity and protection. It establishes to the aggressive individual that they do not have the freedom to victimize anybody who is present at your hospital. In essence, the participants in a show-of-support bear moral witness as well as stand ready to move to act protectively to assist the potential victim of violence or other aggression.

> The show-of-support is exclusively a procedure for **unarmed**, aggressive individuals.

Who Participates in a Show-of-support?

There are four main protocols for a show-of-support. Each has advantages and disadvantages.

All agency. In this case, every staff member of the hospital – clinical, clerical, support, even maintenance – is fully trained and regularly practiced in show-of-support procedures. This only works when training is regularly updated for all employees. Many hospitals find this procedure impossible to set up because of union rules or other conditions of employment that forbid certain staff from participating. In addition, hospitals may also be quite diffident about using nonclinical employees because, if injured, they may claim that participation was beyond both their scope of employ and their training, and that the hospital is, therefore, liable for the injury they suffered.

All medical/clinical/social services staff on the unit. All clinical/social services staff are trained in show-of-support methods. The unit plan ensures that there will always be enough staff available to enact a show-of-support. The biggest disadvantage is that some aggressive individuals assume they can abuse clerical or support staff to get clinical staff's immediate attention.

A dedicated team at the hospital. Certain staff, called by such terms as "officers of the day" are allocated, usually on a rotating basis, to respond to crises as they occur. This requires careful scheduling, to ensure that there is enough staff available on a day-to-day basis. The advantage of this method is that you will have a dedicated team that is trained and used to coordinating together. The disadvantage is that the team can become an elite within your organization that can lead others to abdicate responsibility for de-escalation of their own aggressive patients.

Trained security guards. Security personnel, as individuals and as a team, can be a wonderful resource, but the hospital must ensure that they are properly trained. The facts are that security personnel are rarely trained in effective verbal communication with aggressive individuals.[34] Without this training, their responses can be crude and inept. In many agencies, by the way, security personnel act in concert with other staff. The task for these agencies is to ensure that everyone trains together, so that in an emergency, each knows what to expect from other members of their blended team.

Basic Criteria of a Show-of-support

1. The maximum number of people involved in a show-of-support should be seven. When less than this number is available, the team must adapt so that they can best address some or all of the functions enumerated below. Priority is determined by the exigencies of the situation.

    *   One **Lead**, who is attempting to de-escalate the aggressive or agitated individual.
    *   Up to four individuals who constitute the show-of-support, standing close, usually behind the Lead. One member of this team is the **Organizer** who either calls the team together, or guides them into position.
    *   Phone person, who calls for emergency assistance.
        a. In lower risk situations, this person stands close to a phone to call the standard emergency number (9-1-1 in the United States) if the situation continues to escalate.
        b. In higher risk situations, this person calls the emergency number immediately, gives an address and exact location where the problem is occurring, a full description of the circumstances, what the perpetrator of aggression looks like and is wearing, who is involved in the situation, and if there are any weapons.
    *   If available, a seventh person who is responsible for the "environment." This includes clearing bystanders out of the area, moving furniture and other hazards out of the way if, by chance, the other members (in an inpatient unit, for example) have to restrain the patient. In cases where seven people are not available, the Organizer should assign one person to be "responsible for the environment."

2. Whenever possible, the Lead keeps the lead. In other words, whoever is trying to de-escalate the person should continue to do so. There are, however, exceptions when someone needs to step in and take over:

    *   In many inpatient and hospital settings, the protocol is for clinical staff to step in when support staff is dealing with an aggressive individual. This requires training within the organization so that it is done smoothly and with tact. Otherwise, aggressive patients will assume that the quickest way to talk to a doctor, or other clinical or social services personnel, is to abuse support staff.
    *   The Organizer should step in, tactfully, if the Lead is emotionally overwhelmed.
    *   If the Lead begins to act in an aggressive or unprofessional manner and is too involved to be aware of it, the person present who has authority (be it institutional or the respect of the embattled Lead) should tactfully step in. This requires training and trust. There must be an institution-wide agreement that such intervention will be honored. *Effective training of all*

staff makes this the most rare of occasions. If you do not want someone stepping in this manner, you must ensure that you have fully participated in and understood the centering and de-escalation procedures outlines in the rest of this book. (see next bullet point)

- The Lead should voluntarily hand over the role in certain circumstances. The best "trade-off" of responsibility is that initiated by the Lead rather than when the Organizer sees a situation falling apart and *must* take over. When should the Lead pass the interactive role to another person?

   a. When the Lead is aware that the individual has a special rapport with one person in the vicinity. One must be careful here, however. If one automatically hands the Lead role over to the patient's "favorite" person, your staff can easily be enmeshed in an individual's manipulative game playing. For a "hand over" to occur, the overall situation and everyone's safety must *demand* it. It is not enough that the aggressive individual simply likes someone else better.

   b. The Lead should hand over the responsibility to de-escalate the aggressive individual when they are aware that they are losing their temper or otherwise becoming so flooded or overwhelmed that they can no longer effectively interact with the person.

   c. If the aggressor is <u>absolutely</u> focused on one person as the source of their grievance, and the entire situation is centered around them targeting that particular person, it is sometimes a good idea to remove them from the aggressor's presence.

   d. <u>Inpatient facilities</u> – In many facilities, the charge nurse has ultimate authority and steps in to take over whenever she or he deems it clinically and tactically necessary. This policy should be carefully considered. It can easily lead to a situation where psych techs, para-professionals and other staff abdicate responsibility for verbal de-escalation. Furthermore, the charge nurse may not necessary be skilled in verbal de-escalation either: it is imperative that he or she acquires those skills, and does not merely rely on their professional authority. Inpatient units function far better when all clinical staff have a high level of skill and responsibility in verbal de-escalation.

3. In the event that another party intervenes, the Lead should step back. If they disagree with the intervention, they must do so in a post-crisis staffing after the incident is over. Particularly if the Lead is angry, they will be the last person to acknowledge that they have lost their temper. By definition, anger justifies itself. Nonetheless, <u>the agency requirement must be that if someone "steps in," the Lead "steps back."</u>

Procedures for a Show-of-support

1. The situation starts when the Lead calls for help, or the Organizer, alerted that there is a problem, gathers the show-of-support team.

2. The Organizer is either the first person to become aware of the need for the show-of-support or the person delegated to lead. No matter what the person's position is within the agency, the Organizer's orders must be obeyed (unless, of course, such commands are dangerous or unethical).

3. There should be a maximum of four people arrayed in the actual show-of-support, standing behind the Lead. If there are only four people total available, then three should array in the show-of-support, one always allocated to call your area's emergency number. If there are only three people, or two people, the conditions are the same – one is always allocated to call the emergency number. If there is only one person besides the Lead available, they should first call the emergency number, and then act as needed. Whenever possible, delegate someone to clear the room, and otherwise take "environmental responsibility." If enough team members are available, that should be their only role. In other circumstances, they first lead out vulnerable individuals or other bystanders and then step into the ranks of the show-of-support. One other person may be responsible for the "equipment" – walking restraints, or wrap-around safety blanket (a padded soft-shield, sometimes referred to as a "taco").

Large numbers of people are not helpful.

In fact, the likelihood of intervention to help a victim goes down as number goes up beyond four or five, because there is a diffusion of responsibility – everyone naturally looks to the others around them to know what to do. If you are in a group of ten people, and none of them are moving to intervene, it is very likely that you will not move either. This "crowd inertia" is the cause of many infamous incidents where a person is assaulted or even murdered with a myriad of onlookers standing by, none of them moving to help.

---

4. The team goes to the place of confrontation and lines up. Ideally, they are behind or to the side of their fellow worker. They must not block the exit unless the unit is locked, or the person will present serious risk to others on the other side of the door, and it is your responsibility to keep them safe. When not blocking an exit, it is ideal for your team to angle themselves in such a way that they create an avenue indicating the exit. Do not circle around the aggressive person: not only will they feel surrounded and under attack, but they will also not focus on the Lead. When you encircle the aggressor, you are indicating that you have given up on a peaceful resolution.

5. Each stands with the arms in front, one hand holding the *wrist* of their other arm. One foot should be in front, with the back foot angled somewhat out. Do not stand with your feet in a straight line; the back foot is off to the side. Your faces are blank with your eyes staring distantly, as if you are wearing masks. The members of the show-of-support (other than the Lead, of course) look at the silhouette of the person, not into their eyes.

6. Do NOT stand square – although appearing strong, it is weak. The slightest shove will unbalance you (Chapter 38).

7. Do not clasp your hands. In your nervousness or anxiety, you may begin to wring them.

8. Do not put your hands in your pockets (clueless), behind your back (clueless or hiding something) or cross your arms (confrontational).
   a. Do not simply let your hands hang at your sides. If nervous or tense, you will begin to use your hands in unconscious movements to soothe or discharge tension.

9. The members of the show-of-support team present a united front, demonstrating that their fellow worker is not alone, and that they <u>witness</u> what is going on. They must not verbally respond to the assailant, merely witness. To reiterate, **no matter how provocative the assailant is, no matter what ugly things he or she says, the participants in the show-of-support must not verbally respond. Furthermore, they must not show by their facial expression, muscular tension, or posture that the aggressive person has "gotten" to them.** If a participant does respond, that splits your strength and puts the perpetrator of aggression in control.

10. The Lead continues their verbal de-escalation tactics. Here are the guidelines for the team:

   • You are bearing moral witness ("You will not victimize our fellow worker under our eyes!") and, in some circumstances, you are lining up for possible physical restraint.

   • If the aggressor demands to know why these people are there, why they are listening in or violating his or her privacy, simply say, calmly, "They are just here to keep things safe."

   • If the aggressor attempts to split solidarity by abuse, verbal attacks, or threatening statements and gestures toward the show-of-support participants, the Lead must verbally redirect the individual to them, continuing to try to de-escalate them. The Lead might say, using their name, "Kenneth, you are talking to me." The other members **must not verbally respond.**

   • Remember, direct eye contact on the part of the Lead, blank, almost mask-like faces on the part of the show-of-support. By standing together, you appear organized and trained. This is why everyone should clasp a wrist with the other hand.

What Happens Next?

1. On many occasions, the individual will leave: sometimes quietly, sometimes yelling threats or cursing.

2. In some circumstances, if it is part of your hospital's protocol, the team will shift to physical restraint tactics. These tactics require hands-on training and will not be outlined here.

3. **If the individual attacks the Lead or anyone else, of course, you should assist your coworker. You have a moral responsibility to help protect them.**

4. When police come, one person, either the Lead or the Organizer will brief police on what is happening. Be sure to inform the police clearly what it is you wish to accomplish, be it a trespass warning, simple assistance in calming someone down, getting the person into restraints, reporting a crime, and so on. That said, you must understand that police <u>will</u> take over. It is their job to respond to emergency situations, based on their trained assessment of immediate risk. In many situations, they will take your advice or follow your lead, but in other situations, they will very definitely <u>not</u> do so.

When NOT to Enact a Show-of-support

If the perpetrator of aggression is brandishing a weapon, in particular, a gun, knife or other lethal instrument, staff should <u>not</u> enact a show-of-support. Even a very big, weaponless man or woman can be subdued physically by four or five ordinary-sized people, at least if the latter are intent on stopping the aggressor by any means necessary. This is implicit in the show-of-support, even though you are not standing in a threatening or intimidating manner. This is not really possible, however, if the person has a lethal weapon in their hands. A gun or a knife conveys an almost "godlike" status to the bearer, because they can take life with a single gesture. Therefore, a show-of-support to an armed individual simply offers up your staff as hostages.

To make matters worse, the more hostages, the more dangerous the situation will become. Most hostage takers injure or kill their victims because of heightened anxiety or other stressors. Given that a large group of people is harder to control, the hostage taker may, either panic-stricken or viciously, hurt or murder one of the hostages to control the others. Therefore, the protocol with an armed aggressor is to clear the building or go into lockdown status (doors locked and barricaded). The choice of what to do is driven by your ability to escape. You use lockdown when you can't escape.

As odd as this may sound, escape or lockdown is actually the right way to make the hostage safer. The armed individual, feeling in control, is less likely to attack his or her single hostage, than they would were they to have a group of hostages.

To be sure, there are exceptions to every rule. For example, imagine an enraged twelve year old half-heartedly brandishing a knife. In such a case, staff may decide to remain on site and use a show-of-support, conceivably each holding a chair with legs out to fend off any attack. Consider, too, an inpatient unit, where a patient grabs a syringe, and staff, with nowhere to go and many patients to protect, similarly brandish chairs or mattresses in a coordinated group. However, if staff decide to make an exception, they must be willing to take responsibility for things going wrong. They must be able to clearly enunciate why such an exception clearly seemed in order, whether it worked or not.

CHAPTER 64

The Aftermath:
What to Do Now?

Rage, and, even more so, violence, are an exhausting experience – both emotionally and physically. Many people get the "shakes" after such an incident. So much blood has "pooled" inside the core of their bodies to prepare for combat that they feel cold and start to tremble.

Most individuals have a significantly impaired ability to remember what happened in sequence. One way the sequence gets out of order is they recall the act of defense as the initial attack. They may have a patchy memory of a few events. Much of the rest of the incident is a blur. Although they may be remorseful, they usually do not remember what happened, how it started, or who was responsible.

Even more drastically, they can lapse into a state of defensive confusion where they no longer recall what happened at all, or they completely distort the incident in their memory, thereafter taking no responsibility whatsoever.

Others may feel profound guilt. This might be positive, if it were to lead them to reflect on their own responsibility, but for most people, this guilt is so noxious that they project responsibility onto the person who "makes them" feel so bad. Thus, they soon shift to resentment and begin to blame the other person. Humiliation, the feeling of having one's faults or vulnerabilities involuntarily or forcibly exposed to others, is quite common, and here, too, many people quickly become defensive. Some people have described humiliation like being flayed and exposed. Some respond to shame by becoming enraged all over again. Their thinking seems to be, "If I feel this bad, someone must be doing it to me."

What is almost universal is a post–crisis fatigue, a combination of the depletion of energy stores in the body and the cumulative effect of all the mood and cognitive changes described above.

Taking Care of Your Patient

If the person is still at the hospital after the crisis, your tasks are to maintain control, establish limits and consequences, and possibly regain rapport and provide reassurance, as long as the latter is not a "reward." In other words, you reassure the individual that you are not going to try to get revenge, but neither are you going to pretend that nothing serious happened nor are you going to reward them just because the aggression is over.

If the person is someone who can accept conversation and help after the crisis is resolved, your first responsibility is **clarification**: clearly delineating what you consider abusive, aggressive, or otherwise unacceptable behavior.

If the situation continues to be volatile, if the individual has clearly violated rules or other people's rights, or if safety or tactics demand it, you must go right into **limit setting**. You will inform the person of the severity of what they did, and what the consequences are. Consequences can include anything from being placed in seclusion, being barred from the hospital, being required to leave, or simply being required to sit alone to reflect on what led them to act aggressively. Limit setting and offering consequences must be differentiated from "holding a grudge." The aggressive patient needs to experience consequences for their actions, but we must strive to keep them from experiencing this as punishment or attack. Your tone can have disappointment or outrage, but you are trying to communicate that what they did was wrong, not that they are bad or evil.

If the person is really frightened or devastated by what happened, the first priority is **reassurance and orientation**, letting him or her know that they are not going to be harmed or punished. In cases with people who are experiencing dementia, psychosis, or otherwise in fragile mental states, you may have to let them know what has happened, where they are, what is going to happen, who you are, and so on.

Although **educative follow-up** frequently must be deferred to a later time, individuals who are calm enough to understand should participate in the following:
- Discussing what other tactics they might have used to get what they desired
- Assisting them in becoming aware of patterns that led up to the aggression or assault
- Negotiating agreements on how to avoid such incidents in the future
- Assisting the person to return to a sense of dignity and integrity.

Some people are NOT suited to have such a debriefing. Developmentally delayed individuals or others with dementia or cognitive impairments cannot really remember what happened, and they may re-escalate thinking they are under attack. With people who do not have the mental capacity to really understand the details or implications of what happened, it is better to be calming and reassuring. Other people who can comprehend their actions still need to be left alone for a while to soothe and calm themselves. They need to be spoken to later, not while they are still somewhat escalated.

Consolidation of Gains
Refer to Chapter 3, Consolidating Gains, for more information about how to ensure that your patient learns from the critical incident, and, furthermore, how you can assess if they have learned.

It is not enough, however, to simply reiterate an agreement. For your part, if you have promised some kind of action, let them know clearly what you can do and give them a timetable of when you will do what. If they do not get the results that were promised, they will not only feel betrayed, but they will also be much harder to calm in future disputes.

SECTION X

A Culture of Safety

CHAPTER 65

Establishing A Culture
of Safety

You have read what could have been an entire book about you: your responsibilities to your patients; how to keep yourself calm and centered in chaotic situations; and how to communicate with anguished, confused, and even dangerous people. The weight, however, should not be on you alone. A hospital is a community, and care of patients must exemplify the care society should offer our most vulnerable.

A hospital or residential treatment center should be a haven from the harsh world in which so many of our patients live. Here they may find counsel, treatment of illness, and help in establishing a better life beyond its walls. It should also be a safe haven for us. How can we offer assistance to others, sometimes at a tremendous expenditure of time and energy, if we are looking over our shoulders in fear? A facility that does not protect its own is not in a position to offer the help that people need.

This is not only a concern for staff. How can our patients possibly heal, or even concentrate on their concerns, if they are afraid of being assaulted, having possessions stolen, or having their fragile stability threatened by other patients who are intrusive, manipulative, or disruptive?

An Institution Grounded in Sound Principles

Individual skills are far easier to learn when management has established an ethic in which safety and security are paramount. Far too many people come to harm because they are distracted by other issues rather than focused on what is right in front of them. Although some of the following items may seem far from immediate instructions on how to deal with a frightening or aggressive person, without firm grounding in basic principles, we have nowhere to stand. Here are the elements of a sound safety foundation:

Care. If staff do not believe themselves to be taken care of (adequate safety, benefits, pay), anxiety and resentment will increase, no matter what administrative procedures and rules are in place. Employees who must focus on their own day-to-day survival have far less energy to devote full attention to their patients.

Job security. If staff do not have a sense of job security, anxiety and resentment will increase, no matter how the hospital ostensibly cares for them. Of course, no one is guaranteed a job for life. Nonetheless, when staff trust that management and human resources will take into account such things as outplacement, job search, or other counseling when an unavoidable staff reduction is necessary, they are far more committed to the well-being of the organization. Enhancing job security engenders a sense of reciprocity, where employees are committed to the well-being of the organization and its members, and the organization is equally known to be committed to its members.

Power. If staff do not have a sense that their work and ideas count, anxiety and resentment will increase, no matter what "security" they have. "Security" is a parental level of care, something that any large organization should offer. "Power" means that employees have a voice – not only do they matter as employees, but they are also valued as individuals. If people have concerns or ideas, they have an assurance that what they have to say will be given due consideration.

Respect. If staff do not have a sense that they are treated with respect and dignity, anxiety and resentment will increase, no matter what "power" they have. Staff have a sense that they are not only cared for and even listened to, but also given responsibility and held responsible.

Protection. If staff do not have a sense that they will be protected from violent or threatening individuals, fear and anxiety will increase, no matter how respected they feel. Staff know the agency is proactively working to ensure their safety, as much as is possible. This includes the following:
- Management supports staff when they set limits on verbal violence and harassment, whether it comes from other patients, outsiders (family members, advocates, etc.) or even other staff. Staff know that their concerns will not be minimized.
- Training regarding safety is comprehensive. Practicing skills learned in such training must be agency policy, required at regular intervals.
- Although *violence* on the part of staff would never be condoned, staff have assurance that if they are required to physically protect themselves in a manner that conforms to the law, the agency will provide legal assistance as well as psychological counseling or critical incident debriefing whenever necessary.
- Staff know the avenues for consultation when dealing with a difficult or dangerous situation. Furthermore, they have assurance that the agency will avail itself of outside, expert consultation when resources are not available in-house.
- Staff have confidence that new hires will be fully vetted. If staff members present any risk to anyone, they will be expeditiously retrained or terminated as the situation warrants.

The Essential Factors in Establishing a Safe Worksite
The possibility of aggression on the part of a patient or other individual working at your hospital will be minimized by a number of factors.

Good policy. Policies must be fair and predictable. Patients, even more than staff, must have an assurance that the rules will be the same tomorrow as they are today, and that they will be informed if something must change: be it a schedule, a menu, or an appointment. Many of our patients live in a world of chaos, both with their social environment and what goes on inside their mind. That we, in any way, unnecessarily add to that sense of chaos is the height of cruelty.

Standardization of procedures. Given the fluid nature of human relationships, staff will never be limited in their opportunities for creativity. Nonetheless, there MUST be standardized procedures for dealing with aggressive individuals within the hospital milieu. It is true that you sometimes have to make an exception and go outside the rules, but you must understand that, in doing so, you are taking *personal* rather than institutional responsibility for your action. It may be the right thing to do, but you will have to prove it: not only by positive results, but also by your explanation. In any event, this must be the most unusual of occasions.

Solid boundaries. One subset of predictable and fair rules concerns relationships between patients and staff, staff and other staff, and between patients. Patients must know that staff is vigilant in maintaining ethical and moral relationships between everyone in the milieu.

Everyone needs a sense of privacy to be safe. Therefore, in many settings, patients may not go into each other's rooms. In others, patients may only enter with explicit permission. Invasions of private space are one of the most frequent triggers of violent outbursts

Particularly in psychiatric institutions, patients may not touch each other. Although one patient may believe that they are merely being friendly, hugs, strokes and other physical contact can be perceived as an attack or invasion. Furthermore, some profoundly ill patients may suffer unwanted touch in silence, unable to muster the ability to object.

There must be clear rules regarding borrowing, lending, or giving personal possessions. Antisocial patients will often use leverage or intimidation to get things they want, and disorganized people can forget that they lent their possessions in the first place.

Adaptability. Notwithstanding the necessity for a predictable milieu with standardized procedures, staff must also be flexible. Staffing constraints, a lack of beds, and patients who, for a number of reasons, are disruptive to the unit require immense creativity. Standardization must never become rigidity. An authoritarian, rule-bound unit will engender as much distress among patients as a chaotic one.

Presence and accessibility. The safest units are ones where staff circulate among the patients, *not* those where staff stay behind a barrier or in a room, leaving the patients to mill around unattended. Furthermore, patients need to know their contact person, one staff person on each shift to whom they can speak to and get help. Presence is important for another reason: patients, isolated, can hurt themselves. They can also be hurt or be exploited by other patients. Only when staff are an *active* presence on the unit, aware at all times where patients are, can they keep their vulnerable charges safe. Beyond their physical safety, patients, thereby, have a sense that they are cared for, that your concern is truly for their well-being.

Integrity. Beyond all else, you must embody what you desire patients to be. You must be a person of dignity and integrity. Integrity is perhaps the paramount human virtue. It is closely linked with another virtue – dignity. It is not only our own dignity that we must preserve. As a professionals dealing with some of the most vulnerable members of our human family – people who are often shunned outcasts from both the larger society and, even more tragically, their own families – we are morally responsible to strive to do whatever we can to preserve their dignity.

Above all, be yourself

This should be your greatest strength, but this is only so when you require yourself to offer the best of you to your profession. Without this, all the de-escalation methods in the world are just empty words. The root word for courage and heart, *coeur*, is the same. To de-escalate and calm others requires both.

A Safety Plan

Safety planning is not only the concern of management, security, and clinical staff. You must also include the ideas of clerical and custodial staff, who often have as much or even more face-to-face contact with patients. Don't forget people who may be around less than full time: volunteers, interns, staff who work at multiple sites, lab technicians, and chaplains.

Make sure all employees know the overall plan. In addition, teams within the agency should practice components of the safety plan for which they are responsible. You do not have to practice *everything* – rather, take one element to highlight on regular occasions. You can do this during team or staff meetings. The establishment of a plan must include the following:

A review of the current policies and procedures. Know what is expected at the site where you are working. What practices within the unit might contribute to an environment in which irritation, anger, or even violence is a natural consequence?

- "Let me talk to someone who can actually make a decision!" Consider, for example, if your patients must request services or ask information from one or more people who can't make a decision, thereby forcing them to tell the same story over and over again. It is very important to *minimize layers* for people to get to the person who can actually help them.
- "How can you help me when I don't even know where I am?" Consider a "compartmentalized" institution, bewildering in its complexity. When someone asks for assistance, the usual response is to direct them onward, all too often in the wrong direction. When a person is lost or confused, get up and help them rather than pointing them on their way. If this is the ethos of the entire hospital, staff will save time, and patients and visitors will find themselves more welcomed.
- "Oh, did you call before?" Are calls frequently dropped when people are put on hold? Are they misdirected to the wrong number, requiring them to start over again? Is there a long automated message system with many buttons to push, confusing directions, and no opportunity to talk to a live person for a long sequence of many layers of instructions? All of these are infuriating:

think of the last time you tried to speak to a decision-making individual at your bank or credit card company.

- "Let's start the helping process by humiliating you, shall we?" When there is a multilayered screening process, staff should be trained to ask only the questions necessary to help the person get to the next level. Screening is not therapy, but it can require an equal amount of self-disclosure. Unlike therapy, however, there is no immediate return. When people must answer potentially embarrassing details of their lives over and over again, they may become shamed or angered, thereby damaging any therapeutic effect that could potentially occur when they finally discuss the information with a person possessing the training and authority to do something about the problem. Being required to reveal personal details, only to go to the next level and be asked the same questions over and over again, is humiliating. If certain information is essential, be able to explain clearly why requests for personal information are a necessary component of the screening process. If you cannot clearly explain why it is necessary, maybe you shouldn't be asking.

An emphasis on consultation. While always being fully cognizant of both confidentiality rules and the legal duty to warn of imminent danger, consult with coworkers, supervisors, and in some circumstances, friends and family, about any troubling interchange.

- One type of consultation is a discussion regarding systemic safety concerns. This should not be a "venting" session – rather, it should be a planning session in which you note dangerous issues affecting your unit: a patient's behavior, another unit's or agency's poor reporting of potentially dangerous individuals, or even inadequate lighting in the parking lot. At the same time, one must be realistic. It is not helpful to *problem solve* things that are impossible to change.

- Another form of consultation, usually one-on-one with fellow staff or a supervisor, concerns your patients, particularly after a critical incident. In addition to expressing negative feelings or concerns, you should attempt to understand the situation and see how it developed, and what transition/turning points there were in the intervention. Consultation is an opportunity to get feedback, correction, and advice. Do not hesitate to use consultation due to either embarrassment or pride.

- On other occasions, you need a "fair witness," one or more people who care about you and respect you enough to simply hear you out (see Chapter 27).

A communication system for emergencies

- **Have emergency numbers on the speed dial of your phone**. In addition to the emergency dispatch number (9-1-1 in the United States), this can include the numbers for poison control, child protective services, or the mental health professionals who, in your state or province, are responsible for placing severely mentally ill people in psychiatric hospitals.

- **Whenever possible, use a landline when calling emergency dispatch for help**. In North America, and possibly elsewhere, your address will automatically flash on-screen so that, even when you cannot speak freely, the emergency operator will know where you are.

- **In-house emergency call buttons** that trigger an audible or silent alarm, even including a light over the doorway of the room where the crisis is occurring, are excellent tools. However, installing the buttons is not enough. Your agency should have regular drills to be sure that the alarms actually work and that designated people actually respond when an emergency button is pressed.

- **Develop codes to call for assistance**. Your hospital should have an agreed-upon code word or name that, if used, will activate emergency procedures – a show-of-support, the mustering of security, *and/or* a call to law enforcement. This code phrase can be used over the public address system to summon aid as required.
- **Use code phrases to call for help from your office phone**. It is possible that you find yourself in a situation where you need to call for help but not let your aggressor know that you are doing so. Use the code phrase on the phone, making a request **in context** to the dispute or discussion. *Whenever the agreed-upon name is voiced, no matter what the context of the call is, the recipient knows that the designated safety plan must be initiated.* Note the following examples:
- "Could <u>Mr. Huntington </u>please come here with these records I was talking about? I'm in the conference room. "
- "This is Joanne Newell. Could you please tell <u>Dr. Huntington </u>that I'll be late for my next appointment?"
- "Could you ask <u>Ms. Huntington</u> to call me in room 322? There's a matter regarding hospital policy that I don't really understand."
- "I need an <u>immediate legal consult</u> with <u>Mr. Huntington</u> concerning whether CPS needs to be called when a child is spanked without leaving any bruising."

Some hospitals use a second code to simply call one person down to check out the situation or offer support. Rather than using a fictitious name in this circumstance, I recommend a *code word* to alert the person that the situation is heated and it may be necessary that they stand by, ready to assist in de-escalation or in initiating a show-of-force. In <u>this</u> circumstance, you do not have an emergency – yet. There is, therefore, no need to obscure your intentions from the patient. Instead, you could call the front desk or a supervisor and say, "Mr. DeVore is troubled by our recent phone call to his protective payee. Would you send Ms. Bargetta to this office to *lend a hand* in explaining things to him?" In this case, the somewhat stilted "lend a hand" is used, rather than the more common "help" – and this word is designated, agency-wide, as the code that the situation demands immediate attention.

Examples: Emergency announcements

There are other situations in which everyone must be informed over the PA system, without ambiguity, that they are in an emergency situation. There are two types of announcements:

- A hospital-wide announcement: "Code red on the second floor, east wing. Staff must initiate emergency procedures."
- In other cases, one speaks explicitly: "A man with a gun, wearing a red jacket and brown pants, is in the building. He was last seen on the second floor. Staff must initiate emergency procedures now!" Of course, in situations of such danger, hospitals should use the agreed-upon code to go over the public address system to activate security procedures and inform everyone what and where the emergency is.

Do NOT get beyond the horizon line.[35] Given that you will have many people entering and leaving the hospital on a daily basis, many of whom are unfamiliar, it is imperative that no one "disappears" while on hospital property. Were a staff person to be trapped in a patient's room, in the bathroom, or in a little-used hallway, hours could go by before anyone noticed they were missing. Therefore, check in with each other and let each other know where you are going next.

- "I'm going on rounds. I will be on D wing for about an hour."
- "I'm seeing Mr. Mandell. He's been kind of upset, so please page me in five minutes. If I do not respond, please send security to the room."
- "I'm not feeling well today. I'm going to take a nap in room 423."

Use such contacts as opportunities to do brief co-consultations, or check-in with support staff and other clinicians to find out their observations of your patient while he or she was in the waiting room.

Be aware of who is on your unit. Patients and other outsiders such as visitors must not have the freedom to enter your unit and move around at will, without anyone being aware of where they are and who they are.

Prepare the ground to anticipate a potential problem. There are many situations where an individual or someone connected with them (a parent, an advocate, etc.) must be informed of something that is potentially upsetting, such as being hospitalized against one's will, not being able to return to a former living situation, or losing one's insurance benefits. Discuss the pending situation with other staff and make a plan to prepare for the angry confrontation that might occur. Inadequate staffing or poor planning is a guaranteed formula to kindle people who are already on the edge.

- Plan how best to communicate the disturbing news to the person, based on your *collective* knowledge of him or her.
- Set up the room both in the interests of safety and to best influence their behavior in the way that you desire. This includes making sure that there is an escape route and that there are people in earshot. You might decide to choose a room with warm lighting or soft chairs – or on the contrary, you may choose to select a room that sets a formal tone, where you speak across a table, as if in a business meeting.
- Consider who should be present in the room. (Sometimes the person's counselor, physician, case manager, or family caregiver should be there, and at other times, one or the other of these people should *not* be present.) Sometimes the person closest to the individual is best suited to deliver bad news. In other situations, they should not deliver the news, so that they are viewed as "clean" and still remain as a resource for the person. Base this on the patient's history as well as their current attitude toward various parties.
- Alert staff for the possibility of an emergency and have intervention procedures already set up. In many situations, have someone (security or other staff, depending on your institution) outside the room ready to initiate necessary emergency procedures.
- Be prepared to call law enforcement or security personnel (or have them on site and briefed before you meet the individual of concern).

Review preemptive planning *with* the patient or those associated with them. Certain policies as well as clinical practice often, if unavoidably, upset people. It is often valuable to have such policies CLEARLY explained in written form, which you will review with the patient and have them sign to signify agreement. Enrollees in your program must make an explicit, unambiguous agreement to abide by safety policies. In long-term placement settings, you will need to go over those policies on regular intervals, both to remind the patient of the agreement and to make it clear that you take such agreements seriously. Here are some examples:

- The schedule of activities on the unit, requirements concerning being on time for unit events, and other unit rules must always be absolutely clear to patients.
- Rules regarding sobriety, sexual harassment and other sexual behaviors, and weapons on site, etc., should be clearly explained and placed in writing with the patient required to sign, if he or she is able. Consequences of violating these policies should be clear and unambiguous: If enforcement of such rules is carried out as a "judgment call" at the whim of various staff, manipulative individuals will soon succeed in "splitting" the agency, setting various members at odds against each other. In this case, splitting is not the patient's "fault." It is the fault of the unit and staff who do not universally enforce the rules.
- Furthermore, in institutions such as inpatient psychiatric units, it is sometimes excellent policy to have all the staff sign that they have reviewed and understand the policies and procedures.
- Some individuals, particularly those with strong antisocial traits, should be disqualified from treatment if their purpose for being on a unit is to victimize or intimidate others. We have a responsibility to protect all patients on the unit, and requiring vulnerable individuals to be in the company of those who desire to victimize them is terribly unfair to such patients. Nonetheless, agencies are often required to serve antisocial individuals because of medical needs, by contract, or by some larger agency that dictates policy. <u>Your hospital must set up a rigorous security plan when required to serve such dangerous people</u>.

Adequate staffing patterns. Inadequate staffing can lead to chaos in inpatient units and residential settings. Everyone, staff and patients, will be on edge. Staff members are concerned that they will not be able to attend to problems when they occur. The longer one waits to intervene on volatile situations, the worse they become. Insufficient staffing will lead to a heightened sense of anxiety among your patients. Hospitalized individuals derive a sense of security through an orderly daily routine and kind, firm supervision. Overworked and harried staff often become brusque or too busy to attend to patients' concerns. Finally, due to the lack of supervision in an understaffed unit, manipulative individuals will begin to act in provocative, even predatory ways, particularly toward the most psychologically vulnerable patients.

The question of "group staffing" with the patient

Patients often have a number of people involved in their care, and some hospitals have group meetings with the patient and all caregivers in one room. This might include a therapist, case manager, probation officer, protective payee, child protective services social worker, domestic violence advocate, financial worker, and family members to name only a few. It is possible that if the patient is not caught up in an adversarial relationship with some part of the social services or legal system, such a meeting can be both collegial and productive.

However, such meetings are often called when there is an impasse in a case, or when some type of sanction is being discussed. Although the professionals may believe that they are working in the patient's best interests, the patient often does not perceive it that way. Furthermore, despite the best intentions, the professionals often do not agree on what that "best interest" is or on how to prioritize their competing responsibilities. The social services and medical professionals can overtly, or more often covertly, argue with each other, and this can evoke negative emotions within the patient. Finally, no matter how everyone tries, the patient almost always feels ganged up on. I recommend that this type of case "staffing" be kept to an absolute minimum and only used when all the concerned professionals can clearly enunciate why this serves the patient's best interests.

I recommend that such staffing take place without the patient. Designate someone to get the patient's ideas and bring them to the meeting. Draw up a clear and unambiguous case plan. Assign one person whom the patient trusts, possibly the same one who got their input, to explain the case plan. They are responsible for making sure that the patient fully understands how to implement the plan and who to go for help. In such cases, the plan should be presented in several "media" – explained verbally and drawn out on paper, perhaps with easily followed diagrams, with all phone numbers, addresses, offices, and the schedule and sequence of actions clearly shown.

The patient's input in case planning is paramount. Plans should not be presented as fiat, crafted by a group of professionals behind closed doors. However, team meetings are often a terrible way to assist the person that everyone claims to be helping. They can be intimidating or even overwhelming. Rather than an ideological commitment to "group process," there should be a commitment to setting up the conditions wherein the patient's ideas can best be voiced, and furthermore, that any case plan is presented in a way that offers them the best opportunity to question, contribute, and disagree.

Calling security or the police. Police should be called when anyone is at physical risk or when an aggressive individual is disrupting the activities of your facility. You must give the 9-1-1 dispatcher as complete information as possible, including a description of the aggressor, their current location, whether they have weapons, their current behavior and potential risk. Whenever possible, inform emergency responders of exactly what help you are requesting. You must understand that the police, as emergency responders in cases of potential danger, <u>will</u> take over to establish safety based on *their* assessment of risk at that moment. This may include arrest of the individual of concern.

- Remember, <u>confidentiality rules are suspended</u> in situations of immediate danger. You can speak freely to the police or other emergency responders about your patient in these circumstances.
- One of your most valuable tools is a <u>trespass warning</u>. When law enforcement officers escort a dangerous or undesirable person off the premises, a person whom you do not wish to ever return, request that they be given the "trespass warning." Once this is given, they will be in misdemeanor, or in some cases felony violation, of the law if they re-enter the property, and they can be arrested. Be sure to ask the officer for the case number.

Crisis Intervention Team

One of the most exciting innovations in law enforcement in both America and Great Britain is the CIT – Crisis Intervention Team model, in which law enforcement officers get forty hours of training on dealing with mentally ill individuals in crisis. In many law enforcement agencies, somewhere between 20 to 40 percent of the officers are CIT trained. These are law enforcement officers who work an ordinary shift. However, they are called, whenever possible, when an individual presents somewhere in their jurisdiction with a possibly dangerous mental health crisis.

- Find out if your local law enforcement agency has a CIT team. If they do, ensure that all members of your hospital know about it and what, exactly, such a team can do. If not, lobby to get such training made available.
- If there is a CIT team, always ask for a CIT officer when calling 9-1-1 (or the equivalent emergency number in your country) in crisis situations involving a mentally ill or drug-affected individual. You are not guaranteed a response from a CIT officer: this depends on their availability at the time of the call. Nonetheless, if a team exists, always ask.

Liaison with law enforcement. One way to increase the effectiveness of a working relationship with law enforcement is to offer brief training sessions (for example, on morning watch), regarding some aspect of your hospital and its procedures and responsibilities that would be of value to law enforcement personnel, either in and of itself, or to aid in better liaison with your agency.

It can also be very helpful to discuss problematic individuals who are causing a lot of attention within both systems (for example, an individual who makes chronic suicidal threats or parasuicidal actions). Check with legal advisors in your area to find out your legal requirements and rights regarding discussing patients with law enforcement.

Don't teach police how to do their job

When offering training or consultation to law enforcement, provide concrete information about behaviors of people or about how to access the system. Do not recommend ways for police to "do their job better." Do not talk down to officers, assuming that they have no experience with mentally ill patients . Many police, on a daily basis, have more face-to-face contact with aggressive mentally ill people, particularly at the high end of the spectrum of rage, than most hospital personnel see in a year.

CHAPTER 66

Good Policy,
Good Practice

No matter how skilled you may become at verbal de-escalation, you are dealing with other human beings who may be unable or unwilling to stop themselves from acting violently, no matter what you say or do. Because many situations are best handled by a team, we should avail ourselves of help whenever possible rather than try to solve dangerous situations on our own. To this end, we must create a community in which assistance is a matter of course. But it is not enough to be *willing* to help. Everyone must know *how* to help. You must know, collectively, what to do if things go terribly wrong.

Such preparation has another benefit. If you and your team do not function in a smooth and coordinated fashion, you will find yourselves chaotically trying to improvise what you should have prepared beforehand. When you are focused as an individual and coordinated as a team, you are far more effective in calming the aggressive person.

Units that have a well-coordinated and well-practiced safety plan feel different as well. Potential aggressors:
- See less opportunities to attack
- Find less pretexts to justify an attack, in their mind
- Perceive that behaving badly feels "wrong," the same way it feels out of place to raise your voice in a museum or church

Preparing for the worst makes it less likely to happen.

Record Keeping as It Pertains to Violence and Risk

Good record keeping is crucial to safe and effective patient care. Clear, concise, and *legible* case notes are essential to the safety of your fellow staff members, who may at times have to work with the patient in your absence. Critical information should be highlighted in a manner congruent with your hospital's policy in the case of handwritten records, so that anyone opening the file is immediately aware of the risk factors involved.

Handwriting is not an issue in agencies were electronic databases are used. However, critical information should be noted on the face page of the patient's electronic file, either through the use of a color-coding system or a visible "alerts" tab.

Any staff person who will be working with an unfamiliar patient should take a few minutes to review their case file, noting any special conditions or alerts contained therein. In fact, all staff should take a moment to review their patient's case file before conducting an interview to remind themselves of previously noted information.

Every patient's chart should have a red divider in the back of the most recent file that includes copies of every known critical incident. If records are computerized, you should have a pop-up screen that serves a similar function. You can, thereby, find similar incidents that may have led a person to be aggressive in the past. Through this, you will be able to discern patterns that help in predicting future incidents. Often, it is *only* when all the incidents are placed together that one is able to see a pattern to the aggression.

Examples: Incidents revealed through record review

- **A woman with borderline personality disorder has aggressive outbursts toward staff.** A review of critical incidents reveals that all her outbursts are at the staff with whom she has, otherwise, the best rapport. When this is brought up to the patient, she reveals that her husband physically abuses her son, and she is reminded of her father abusing her and her brother, while her mother did nothing to stop the violence. She is enraged at staff at the hospital who "should be" stopping the current abuse, something that, in fact, they could not do as she had not disclosed it.

- **A resident at a group home has assaulted staff on three separate occasions on Mondays.** It seems he has family visitation on Sundays, and occasionally, his parents bring his younger brother who continues to be competitive, even though the resident is clearly suffering from mental illness. The younger brother, aged nineteen, teases, demeans, and provokes the patient. Assaults have occurred the day after such visits.

- **On two occasions, a patient admitted to an inpatient unit, after several hours of peace, has suddenly burst into rage, accompanied by an undifferentiated attack, flailing arms and legs, and guttural utterances.** A history review shows that he was a heavy user of PCP. There is evidence that even after a long time of sobriety, some individuals can suddenly have a flashback, as if they have a history of intoxication with this drug. This may be related to heavy exertion. Staff finds that the patient believes exercise is the key to his sobriety, and both flashbacks occurred after a period where he was heavily exercising in his room.

Training and Practice

It is your professional and moral responsibility to be well versed and skilled in de-escalation methods. This certainly requires an effort on the part of the individual, but even more so, it must be agency policy that good training is made available to you, and that times are set aside on a *regular* basis to practice these skills.

Training specific to physical restraints

If restraint procedures are part of the requirements of your job, you must practice them regularly until they are "pseudo-instinctual": a trained response as natural as driving your car or combing your hair. Furthermore, you must maintain an optimum level of physical fitness. Untrained and unfit staff who are responsible for the physical well-being of patients whom they must restrain are dangerous to the patients they are responsible for protecting. Here is a simple assessment of physical fitness as it pertains to physical restraint techniques.

- Clasp a 40- to 50-pound bag of rice in your arms and walk 30 paces, and return 30 paces.
- Without pause, lower yourself to your right knee five times in succession, then to your left knee five times.
- Without pause, raise one foot and balance on the other, still clasping the bag of rice. Reverse and do this with the other.

If you are not able to do this, you are NOT in the proper condition to do physical restraint techniques. Sooner or later, you will surely be hurt. Even worse, you will likely injure patients.

Confidentiality and HIPAA

If the acquisition of the information covered in a release of information is within the scope of your professional responsibilities, then the following section is important.

If the patient refuses to sign a release of information, something they have a perfect right to do, remember that you will not be allowed to share specific details about their progress with others, nothing prevents you from listening to the observations from third parties.

Ask for a release of information at least several times during the course of treatment. Patients are often only asked upon intake when they are most guarded and anxious. Particularly in long-term placements, relevant staff should not refrain from asking again at a later time. In many cases the patient feels more comfortable as a relationship develops and might be more inclined to sign the form.

How to Assess Your Personal Work Space for Danger

Consider your office space. Look at it just in terms of aesthetics. Do you like it?

Confidentiality and information sharing

In most states, there are rules stipulating when collaboration and sharing of information between different agencies is a **requirement**. Check with legal advisors in your locale to find out your legal requirements and rights in your jurisdiction.

NOTE: There are sometimes conflicts between Federal HIPAA laws, and individual state and local laws and ordinances governing confidentiality. Consult with your legal advisor to ensure that you are fully in compliance with the laws governing confidentiality, as well as being able to hold others to those same statutes.

Are you happy to be there? If you are not, perhaps your patients will not be either.

Look at it in terms of a work space. How convenient are things to reach? Consider it now in terms of security: do you have a safe place to lock things away, including patient files and personal possessions?

Now consider it from the point of safety. Think about various journal or magazine articles that you may have read that tell you what items NOT to have in your office space. This can get a little overwhelming, can't it? Just about anything that a person can pick up in one or two hands could be used to hurt another person. How, then, can we make our offices safe and secure?

How neat are your office and your desk? This is not as farfetched a question as you might imagine. A neat office is one in which the owner takes interest. You are staking it out as territory, as clearly as a bear scratching his claws high on the trunk of a tree. A messy, disorderly office gives many people an indication that it is not your territory. Why?
- Your space appears to be owned by no one, and is, therefore, up for grabs.
- Your space seems to show you as someone not in control of your environment.
- Your space seems to reflect that you don't care about the conditions in which you work.
- Your space doesn't embody the kind of life you are encouraging your patients to reach for. As so many individuals who go to social services agencies struggle to establish order in their own lives, we should, at minimum, show it in our own.

Beyond how neat your office should be, your work space should reflect your aesthetic sense. People should get a sense of who you are simply by being there, without there being any disclosure of your personal life.

Establish an escape route. Go through your office/work space and figure out the best escape route from each room. If a crisis is developing, you should try to stand or sit nearest to the exit. For offices that, due to a variety of circumstances, one could not easily escape from, you must also figure out the best way to barricade yourself within. Any limitations (a door without a lock, a flimsy hollow door, windows that are painted shut) should be noted and, whenever possible, corrected. If a door does have a lock, <u>support staff should have keys</u> so that a patient cannot lock himself or herself in the office with a staff person.

Arrange a safe office

- Desks should have at least one locked drawer.
- Put away objects – potential weapons – that are not REQUIRED for the regular function of your job. In other words, things you do not need most of the time (scissors, letter openers, etc.), should be locked away.
- Lock away all personal information. This presents a problem in states where you are required to display a license that has your home address. Secure a mailing address from which you do business. This can be a personal mailbox, for which you use a street address.
- Secure any photos of your family. In addition to being a target of any predatory individual or potential stalker, you may be perceived by some people as flaunting your good fortune in their face. Your good fortune is perceived as a personal attack. To be sure, there are occasions where showing someone, even a patient, a picture of your family is beneficial. However, you should know why you are doing this and what benefit is likely to accrue. If you cannot do so, keep your good fortune to yourself.
- Items that are necessary – that you use on a regular basis – can be on your desk, but whenever possible, not within your patients' immediate reach. Your goal is <u>not</u> to sanitize your work space. It is to mindfully choose what belongs in your office for you to accomplish your job while considering your own and other's safety.

Decide where to place your chair. It seems there is a never-ending question of where to place one's chair. Here are the advantages and disadvantages of each choice:

- Place your chair closer to the door. This provides you with the ability to leave your office expeditiously, but has two disadvantages: 1) your patient can feel trapped, with you blocking the door, and 2) if you want to tell your patients to leave your office, they have to go past you, which can escalate the confrontation.
- Place your patient's chair is closer to the door. Your patients are less likely to feel trapped and enclosed, and they can walk right out if they are requested to leave, but it can conceivably lead to a situation where they block your exit.
- Be flexible. Ideal chair placement can vary from patient to patient: with your 10 a.m. patient, you might want to be closer to the door, while with your 11 a.m. patient, you might want to place him closer to the door.

In sum, there are advantages and disadvantages to both options. You should choose the option that makes you most comfortable, considering the risk and benefits of each.

How to Enter a Room to Ascertain If There Is a Problem and How to Extricate Your Coworker

Let us imagine that you hear loud or threatening voices coming from an office, cubicle, or conference room. Enter the room with a knock on the door and apologize for interrupting. Particularly if the situation looks dangerous, use almost "over-the-top" drama in your apologies. You are trying to "take over" the room without acting aggressive or domineering: "I am so sorry to interrupt you! You know I *wouldn't* dream of doing this if it wasn't important!" Turning to the patient, say, "I'm very sorry. This will only take a moment." Then, create an excuse to draw your coworker out of the room. Here are some examples:

- Ask for the location of a chart, underscoring how urgent this is and how unique and important a situation this is that you would interrupt a session or meeting.
- Ask to consult with your coworker on a problem. Again, with some drama, underscore how important this is, apologizing to the patient for interrupting what is clearly an important meeting of his or her own.
- Tell your coworker that he or she is needed briefly to attend to a small family emergency (i.e., their nephew got a cut at the day care and they need a phone authorization to stitch it up). Make it the kind of "emergency" that can't be easily proven false but that *must* be attended to right away.
- Apologize again as you usher your coworker out.

To the person who might need assistance
- You should already have any personal information locked up in your desk or, in the case of a purse or briefcase, in your hands as you leave.
- Go down the hall out of range of the patient and discuss the situation. If there is no emergency, thank your fellow staff member for trying to protect you. If there is a dangerous situation, act effectively to solve it.

Do NOT
- Refuse them in the presence of the patient. Rather, get up and leave the office and discuss things out of earshot.
- Do not contradict them: "I've never heard of that chart," or "I don't have a nephew."
- Do not berate your coworker who, with your safety in mind, may have interrupted a difficult but productive moment in your work with the patient. Rather, thank them, reassure them, return, and pick up where you left off.

If your coworker is overly anxious or has a "hero" complex and intervenes when no help is needed, give them thanks for their concern, assure them that there is nothing to worry about it, and return to your session, and later take it up with your supervisor as a training issue.

CHAPTER 67

Safety and
New Employees

General Program Issues

It is absolutely essential to make clear to new employees that a culture of safety and nonviolence is a primary focus of your hospital. Therefore, include your newly hired employees in the following:

- Meetings concerning patients who present risk.
- The *regular* trainings in show-of-support (Chapter 63) that your hospital should be holding.
- Instruction on how to set up a safe work space, which should be reviewed by a supervisor.
- Familiarization with all emergency policies. One training/supervision session should go over these procedures. The supervisor should verify that the new employee fully understands and can enact these procedures.
- Signing a written form that gives assent and attests to full understanding of safety policies and procedures.
- Voicing any concerns, and directing all "what should I do if . . ." questions to the supervisor, trainer, and/or safety officer, so that they feel fully prepared to work.
- Clearly understanding that the ethos of the hospital is to ask for supervisory advise whenever you are (1) not sure of something, (2) frightened, or (3) finding yourself off-center or angry due to an interaction with a patient.
- Mentoring with seasoned employees, should be a primary ethos of the agency. Senior staff are expected to make themselves available to assist new employees regarding safety issues.
- Have senior employees or supervisors sit in on their sessions – not only to give advice on their social or clinical work, but also to give advice regarding actions that enhance or impair safety. This, formalized as a mentoring relationship, is invaluable

All of the above applies to nonclinical staff as well. Clerical and support staff often have a more front-line role with patients, at least when the patients first walk into the hospital. Therefore, they are the first to assess risk with a presenting individual and often bear the full brunt of aggression in its initial stages. Training regarding safety, appropriate to the professional responsibilities of nonclinical staff, should be as extensive as for clinical staff. The ethos of respect, in which staff should always feel free to express concern or misgivings, equally applies to nonclinical staff. It is essential that they, too, have a full voice.

Preparing for Problems that Might Happen Before a Newly Hired Person Is Fully Trained

- One of the dilemmas facing agencies is that people can be hired between scheduled safety trainings. The basic information outlined above, however, can and should be presented one-on-one.

- Staff can be quickly trained in show-of-support (Chapter 63) procedures, because they do not require verbal de-escalation skills. As any hospital using show-of-force strategy should be having a weekly or bi-weekly drill in the procedure – different units can do this in five minutes, as part of staff meetings – they will quickly get up to speed.

- Staff can easily be trained to direct people to clear an area. You should use role play practice to do this until you are sure that they can express themselves with tactful, strong authority. This is also a very quick way to begin to assess the capacity of your new staff people to handle themselves in crisis. If you cannot step into a situation and take authority, you cannot solve a crisis.

- Newly hired staff should also be taught how to properly call 9-1-1 (or the equivalent emergency number in your country).

- They should be taught and then expected to alert other individuals within your hospital when an emergency is occurring, including notifying them to escape or lockdown.

- Whether staff have sophisticated de-escalation skills or not, there are two items that they must learn right away that will carry folks through most situations: 1) The agency's safety policies and procedures, and 2) how to center and calm oneself in crisis (Section IV). Centering procedures should be taught as part of orientation.

CHAPTER 68

When Monitoring Medication
is Part of Your Professional
Responsibilities

Make sure that the prescribing physician knows what other medical conditions the patient has, as well as other medications (prescription, over-the-counter, and herbal) that the person is taking. You must be aware of what the intended effect is of each drug, and how the various medications might interact. Furthermore, you must be informed what to look for should the medications have a negative effect on the patient. If you notice that the drug is not having the hoped-for results, speak to both the patient and other members of their treatment team. We sometimes only know that a medication is not suitable when the patient begins to do poorly. This can be a life-threatening issue.

If monitoring patients' medications is not part of your responsibilities, you must, nonetheless, notice if their behavior or symptoms have changed and consider the possibility that they are having trouble with a drug, either prescribed, over-the-counter, or illicit, and urge them to see their doctor. Whenever possible, contact their physician yourself if you believe that there is an emergent issue.

Why Do They Stop Taking Their Psychiatric Medications?

Patients can experience unpleasant side effects. There are very good reasons for people to resist taking their medications, discontinue them, or take them intermittently. Among possible side effects are muscle spasms, intolerable itching/crawling sensations in the limbs, tongue thrusting, tremors, impairment of sexual functioning, dry mouth, weight gain, weight loss, skin disorders, even life-threatening disorders that must be monitored through such invasive procedures as regular blood draws, to name but a few.

Many psychiatric medications are not "felt" beyond their side effects. They do not make the person "high" or even "better." In fact, apart from the side effects, the person simply feels like "himself." Feeling good, therefore, they draw the natural conclusion that the drug has done its job – or in other cases, doesn't work – and therefore can be discontinued.

Even apart from noxious side effects, the illness can feel better than the "cure." Many individuals diagnosed with manic-depressive illness experience a well-medicated, stable life as a terrible sacrifice. Yes, one doesn't get into as much trouble, but from the perspective of the person experiencing mania, one sacrifices life as a skylark for that as a ground sloth. Many individuals experiencing psychotic symptoms find that the medications muffle or suppress delusions and/or hallucinations, but they do not make them disappear. Furthermore, the medications often do not touch the belief system around a person's delusions. Medicated life for such people is like living under a sodden blanket. What is reality to them may be muffled and tranquilized, but not otherwise changed. The medications may help them live a more stable, uneventful life, but just as we shake off constricting bedding when we are too hot and constricted, they may discontinue medications, simply to have, in their view, air to breathe. If you believe your perceptions are real and all the medications do is muffle and obscure that reality, then it is quite natural to discontinue them.

What Should You Know About Your Patient's Medications?

If you are directly responsible for monitoring your patient, what, ideally, should you know about their medications?

- Name of medications (generic and brand name)
- Date prescribed
- Expiration date of prescription
- Number of refills
- Purpose of the prescription
- Side effects that the medication can cause
- Side effects that the person is experiencing
- Palliative measures taken to deal with side effects
- Potential drug interactions between medications
- Actual drug interactions and how they are medically being dealt with
- History of discontinuing medications
- Past reasons for discontinuing medications
- What reasons the patients can give that would lead them to discontinue medications
- Your observations of the effects of the medications
- Based on your experience, can you think of some other helpful pieces of information?

A medication log that lists the drugs that were prescribed can help keep you informed about your patient's pharmaceutical treatment. For maximum effectiveness, the log should not only list the drugs by name but also when they were prescribed, what each medication is for, what side effects to watch for, and your observations on how the medications are affecting behavior and thought processes of your patient. The medication log needs to be kept in a specific part of their chart for easy access during an emergent situation.

CHAPTER 69

Conclusion

The graph below depicts the various tactics I described as they apply throughout the cycle of aggression.

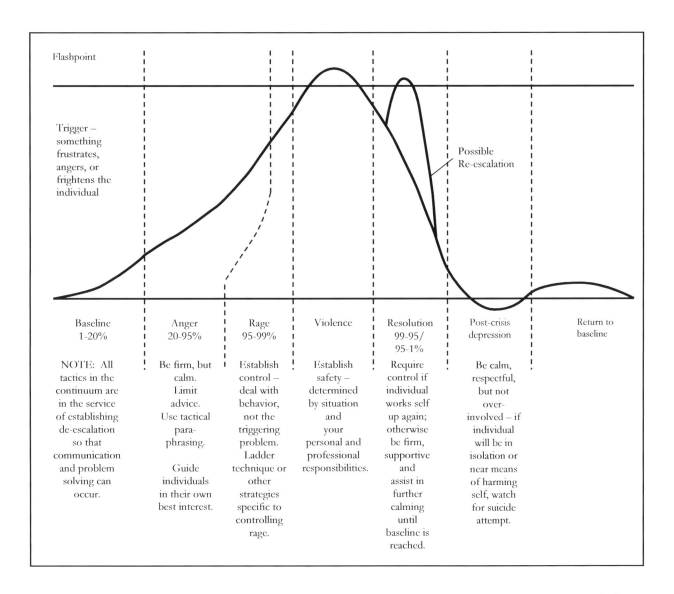

Now that you have finished this guidebook, you have really just begun. It is important to regularly review and update the information in your patients' crisis files. It is equally important that you regularly review and practice the safety and de-escalation methods in this book. You should be as familiar with this information as you are with the information necessary to drive your car or use your telephone. Just as you automatically snatch your hand away from a hot stove, or blink your eyes when a small object flies toward them, these skills must become so familiar to you that they become as automatic as instincts.

It is difficult for many of us to consider the subject of potential violence. It can be so painful to realize that people, at times, want to hurt, or even maim or kill you that you might prefer to pretend to yourself that it isn't happening. Aggression, unattended, hurts everyone far more. Skill in the de-escalation of aggression, and furthermore, establishing a culture of safety within the organization you work, will create a sense of spaciousness that makes you a far better doctor, nurse or social services specialist. Your patients are the ones who will benefit most.

APPENDIX I

A Sample Case Plan for a Patient Who Made Serious Repeated Parasuicidal Attempts

Shauna was in a terrible cycle. Somewhat developmentally disabled, with borderline personality disorder, she was in a mental health program that used a "nurturing model." In other words, the counselors believed that if they were supportive and accepting, Shauna and the other women in the program would do best. For that reason, they "encouraged, but never directed." Among the things they encouraged Shauna to do was to have more of a social life.

Shauna lived in a rough area of town, but following her counselors' suggestions, as best as she understood them, she began going out to bars near her apartment. Naïve, childish, and insecure, she was perfect prey for predators. A man would approach her, speak nicely to her, and suggest they go somewhere private. She'd invite him back to her apartment, where she would be raped. After the attacker left, in each case, she would cut her wrists, deeply, and then call 9-1-1 for help. Even though this happened on a number of occasions, no investigation was successful. She couldn't describe her attacker, except in terms such as, "He was a nice man. He had blonde hair. Why did he do that?"

Because of her childlike nature, most people remained kind. The police talked gently to her, as did EMT. She was taken to the hospital, where the nurses, doctors, and social workers took care of her; a "rape victim advocate" helped her through the rape kit and the fruitless investigation. Then, she would be seen by a mental health outreach worker.

Her therapists gave her emotional support and worked on her "trauma issues." No one told her to stop going to bars, although her therapists and case managers did make suggestions on "being careful," words that meant nothing to Shauna who trusted and acted upon her immediate feelings.

One day, a coworker and I were discussing the case, and we essentially came to the conclusion that we, in the system, had become part of Shauna's rape cycle. Each time she would go to the bar with high hopes of meeting someone, she would be violated and then cut her wrists, *requiring* that a number of kind, strong, wise people would encircle, care for, and comfort her.

We couldn't stop her from going out, we couldn't move in with her to stop the rapists, but we could, without violating any ethics, respond differently. Our perspective was to create the most compassionate possible response from each representative from different parts of the emergency response system, compassion defined as that which would help Shauna no longer be raped.

Here, in brief, was the plan:

- **Police response**. Response time and attempt to investigate the crime was unchanged. However, each officer was to have a flat affect, a nearly emotionless "just the facts" approach to their interview with Shauna. They should not be cold, mean, punitive, or sarcastic. They should simply take the factual information.

- **EMS**. Emergency medical care was unchanged. However, there should be no comforting voice or gesture, no matter how much Shauna was crying or wailing. They should move her to the gurney like moving a sack of potatoes.

- **ER**. Medical treatment unchanged. Anesthesia – of course! – was used when stitching her wounds. (Despite any imputation to the contrary, we were NOT punishing her. We were also not rewarding her.) The doctors and nurses, however, asked no questions beyond what was needed for medical treatment. The social worker, too, would take just the basic facts. If she needed something to drink, she would receive water, not juice or anything sweet. "Sweet" means nurturance – we did not want to nurture her into being raped and possibly getting killed, or killing herself afterward.

- **Rape victim's advocate**. As might be imagined, these big-hearted people, doing a job that few of us could handle, had the hardest time with the plan. With sufficient discussion, however, they understood. Their approach was to be "distantly kind." In other words, the same kind of approach one uses with a child who skins her knee: you tend to her and send her on her way.

- The **emergency evaluator for mental health** would do a full assessment. There would, however, be no counseling, in the sense of emotional support or investigation of feelings, beyond what was necessary to determine if she needed to be hospitalized that night. If Shauna was not immediately suicidal, she was sent home. (This, by the way, was always the case. She would slash herself after the assault for two reasons: It provided endorphin relief from terrible stress, and it was a guaranteed method of getting people to come to her house and give her emotional support. However, she would not do it a second time related to the same incident.)

- **Welfare check**. She would get a call once daily from the crisis line that was kept brief. She would be reminded to see her therapist, and when her appointment was.

- **Counselor's responsibility**. The counselor, at scheduled meetings, would have Shauna go through everything she did that night in exhaustive detail. In a sense, it was an "after-action review," not emotionally rewarding in the least. On the flip side, once this was complete and better safety planning was done ("Don't go to bars anymore," for example), they would talk about other things, and Shauna would get *emotionally rewarded* for non-pathological discussions, thoughts, and actions. The idea is that Shauna would get no emotional reward for suicide or dangerous actions, and *much more* reward for healthy behaviors.

Several weeks subsequent to the implementation of this plan, Shauna again made a suicide attempt after a sexual assault. Everyone held to the plan, although some later confessed that they felt like brutes, seeing this stitched-up child in an adult's body, her clothing blood soaked, walking out of the ER, sobbing like her heart was broken. Her counselors, who were central to any success, began to work with her according to the plan. They learned to provide strong emotional reward for the most mature behaviors that Shauna displayed. In the past, these behaviors were ignored, because they didn't cause anyone any trouble. Shauna began to thrive on being treated as a responsible human being. Rather than having her feelings hurt, she welcomed advice on how to dress and how to live her life. For a period of over fourteen years, she has continued in the same mental health agency, but she has had no contact whatsoever with law enforcement or the emergency medical system, nor has she suffered from any more sexual assaults.

APPENDIX II

Frequent Precipitants
of Violence in
Inpatient Facilities

How this list was compiled

I compiled this list after working for over a decade with two psychiatric evaluation and treatment units in the state of Washington. Every six months, I offered training in verbal de-escalation and physical restraint. We started every training with a check-in in which we would discuss problematic situations that arose in the last six months. These were the most common issues associated with anger and rage among patients.

- Involuntary sanctions or placement
- Arguments about medication compliance
- The termination of services or end of placement
- Transitions – bedtime, mealtime, wake-up, shift changes
- Change – in environment, routine, roommate
- Chores
- Boredom
- Problems with roommate
- Threats from other patients or residents
- Rule enforcement
- Lack of consequences
- Vague or inconsistent rules
- Rigid, excessive rules
- Poor boundaries
- Money disputes
- Entitlements – arguments about entitlements – a sense of entitlement
- Lack of staff training or skill
- Too much unstructured time
- Broken promises
- A chaotic environment with too much noise and stimulation
- A lack of opportunity or choices
- A lack of privacy

- A complicated / passive-aggressive / unresponsive system
- Character problems on the part of staff – being intimidating, withdrawn, impatient, rude, angry, or burned out
- Contact with family, or lack of contact with family
- Holidays, anniversaries, birthdays
- Upsetting news

APPENDIX III

───────

Safety in the
Emergency Room

Emergency rooms present special problems. Unfortunately, this is not because there is a special client population that visits the emergency room. Those in emergency rooms will, if confronted by an aggressive client, use the same strategies of verbal de-escalation and control that they would use in another setting.

The dangers lie in another direction – systemic and environmental. Here I will delineate the dangers and offer one simple suggestion for what to do.

The Dangers

In many states, law mandates or convenience dictates that individuals in psychiatric emergencies are taken to the nearest emergency room, whether or not that facility is equipped for any psychiatric emergencies, and further, is ready to manage assaultive individuals. The problems include the following:

No safe place for the patient. Quite frequently, the patient is left in a room full of weapons of opportunity – sharps, syringes, and any number of items that can be used as bludgeoning instruments or projectile weapons. With startling frequency, suicidal patients are left unattended with full access to a huge variety of items: medication and cutting instruments that they can – and occasionally do – use to attempt suicide. Many hospitals do not have a seclusion room where the patient can both rest safely and be secured.

Understaffed for emergencies. Many smaller emergency rooms are understaffed at night. There are not sufficient individuals at smaller hospitals to assist in, for example, restraint procedures if needed. Many hospitals give their staff no training whatsoever in this area.

No security staff. Many smaller hospitals do not have any security personnel.

Poorly trained security staff. Many smaller hospitals have a single security officer who has no training whatsoever in communication with mentally ill or intoxicated individuals. Their interventions have, on occasion, exacerbated a situation rather than calming it down.

Disempowered security staff. I am aware of one major hospital that has a rather large security force. However, they are forbidden to physically intervene with disruptive patients, and when called, are required merely to stand and observe. Reportedly, the hospital is concerned regarding liability issues.

An interpretation of patient rights that puts staff at risk. Many hospitals, whether staffed by security or not, will not or cannot search patients for weapons or drugs. There have been incidents of patients using either of these items for a suicide attempt or assault.

In many states, due to inadequate beds in both the mental health and drug/alcohol treatments systems, many involuntarily committed patients are literally being "boarded" in the emergency rooms for an entire 72-hour hold. Patients are thereby not getting the clinical treatment they need, and they definitely present with severe management problems in an already over-stressed setting.

Inadequate screening. Particularly with intoxicated or otherwise difficult-to-manage individuals, there is, frequently, an inadequate risk assessment. The patient is both demanding and obnoxious or otherwise hard to communicate with, and this, paradoxically, can lead to less assessment rather than more. A proper risk assessment should include a history of violence and suicide. Particularly with long-term patients in the "system," this information should be immediately accessible to emergency personnel – confidentiality laws being suspended in emergent situations. Procedures need to be in place through which hospital and/or mental health personnel execute a "one-touch" or "one-call" access to information regarding violent history.

Inadequate resources. When an individual does not meet criteria for what should be the least-restrictive alternative, both mental health and hospital personnel have few alternative referrals. This leads to patient and family outrage, and/or the crisis continuing to fulminate until the patient truly presents an unmanageable risk. Examples include these:

- **Detox.** Many detox facilities refuse to take dual diagnosis patients, particularly when their mental health issues, whatever the etiology, are severe. Although allegedly secure settings, many detox units do not have locked units, and the staff have little training or skill in dealing with mental health issues. When the detoxing individual, often with an antisocial history, is then placed, by default, in a psychiatric inpatient unit, they present severe risks to both staff and patients, particularly because they are not receiving treatment appropriate to their condition.

- **Developmentally disabled individuals and other cognitively impaired patients**. All too frequently, a long-term patient in a group home or other facility gets out of control – even violent. There are very few options for such individuals if the care facility decides, rightly or wrongly, that they cannot manage them. In many communities, a very confused, frightened individual, sometimes angry and developmentally disabled, head injured, or suffering from senile dementia, is then brought to the emergency room and evaluated by a mental health professional who has no options for a clinically appropriate referral. Such individuals are often placed, by default, in an evaluation and treatment facility or psychiatric hospital, where their needs are not met. Furthermore, the group-care facility, all too often, may refuse to take the patient back, and, at the same time, does not take responsibility to find the individual a facility that more adequately meets their needs. The mental health professional is placed in an often insoluble dilemma: does he or she commit such an individual who does not have a mental disorder, to a psychiatric facility, simply to keep them safer than they otherwise would be? Or does the mental health professional or social worker insist on sending them back to a facility that is hell-bent on discharging them – at any cost?

In conclusion, then, unless systemic issues are addressed, mental health professionals of all categories may find themselves at particular risk when attempting to assist a patient in an emergency room setting. What should be, in fact, the *most* secure community setting, is, in fact, often among the least.

APPENDIX IV

Managing Threats
to Your Family

More horrifying than any threats to ourselves are threats to our family. The aggressor creates a sense of utter helplessness, promising to attack when we are not there. The threat is usually empty, made in the heat of the moment as means of additional defiance, or meant to terrify. You must, however, take any such threats seriously, because it is almost impossible to know when the threat is real or not. And, truth be told, a bit of preventative planning, and educating family members about being mindful and aware, is never a bad thing.

You must inform your family of threats and of the need to take protective action. In regards to your children, it is your responsibility to explain everything they need to know, but no more. <u>Do not over-explain</u>. Furthermore, if you excessively display your own fears, you will weaken your family members as they become preoccupied with your needs or overly anxious, unable to calmly but safely go about their lives. Remember, a calm strong individual is best able to evaluate dangerous situations. You will also appear less vulnerable to the predatory individual.

It is not enough to simply set up a safety plan. Review your safety plan with your family on a regular basis. If your family is threatened, take action:

Inform law enforcement and get detailed advice on how best to keep your family safe. The investigating officers will assist you in drawing up a safety plan as well as considering what, if any, action they can take on your behalf.

Review home security. Consult with your local police on how to make your home more secure. Some agencies will be more willing than others to send out an officer to walk through and around your home to inform you of security gaps. There are also excellent books on making your home safer. Consider a home alarm system: I would recommend researching with some nonpartisan consumer organizations (i.e., Angie's List, Consumer's Report), as there is a wide variety of quality and price in this field.

The question of owning a gun. Almost anyone can buy a gun. It is the height of irresponsibility to purchase a weapon if you do not intend to acquire extensive training in how to use it safely. If you are buying firearms for protection, you <u>must</u> get training in using a weapon for self-defense. This is a field rife with scam artists and incompetents. Consult with local police agencies for trustworthy training agencies. They should be vetted as extensively as you would vet a babysitter who is going to be responsible for many weeks of care of your small child. Owning and using a weapon is a deadly-serious business, and you and your family should only undertake this with gravity and care.

Dogs for protection. Some dogs, in many ways, are a far better protective agent than a firearm. Unlike humans, they will not hesitate when they perceive a threat. There are several kinds of dogs to consider. Some dogs are not known for their ability to be physically protective, but they will bark vigorously at any intruder, providing you with an early warning system. Others –the Cane Corso (Italian mastiff) is a good example – are loving to their family, particularly children, and naturally protective. They are also BIG. Finally, there are wonderful, intelligent animals such as the German shepherd, who, in addition to a natural protective capacity, can be well trained. On the other hand, raising and keeping a dog is a tremendous responsibility. In essence, you have a child who cannot grow up and for whom you must be responsible. The dog deserves love and care in return for their love and care of you. Further discussion of dog breeds and training is well beyond the scope of this book, but dogs can be one of the most important aspects of a personal protective system for your family.

Are you a soft target or a hard target? A soft target is easily accessible, predictable, and unaware of danger. A hard target is not easily accessible, not predictable, and security conscious. A security conscious person is aware and in touch with his or her surroundings. This is not merely a task for you alone. This is a task for your family as well. To this end, two books by Gavin de Becker are strongly recommended: *The Gift of Fear* and *Protecting the Gift*.[⊠]

Watch your back. You and your family must learn to scan your surroundings to become aware if you are being watched or stalked. Remind family to report suspicious people and cars. You can make this a game with your children – but not as an "under-the-radar" trick. The children should understand why they are being asked to do this – but this does not preclude your making it a challenge or even fun. Ask them to notice people and tell you if they see them again elsewhere. Ask them if they have ever seen someone – maybe wearing different clothes – on another occasion or location. Ask them to count cars while driving or play "slug bug" (calling out Volkswagens), but in addition, to tell you if they see a car over and over again.

Make sure your family's work and school settings are **aware of the identity of the potential assailant**.

Both you and your family should **change routines** on a daily basis. Travel by different routes at different times. Don't always go to the same store, the same coffee shop, and so on. Be unpredictable.

Don't be alone. Neither you nor you family should be the last person to lock up or leave a work or school location. Enlist coworkers, coaches, school personnel, and others to be part of a team.

Whom to trust. Make very clear to those involved with your children who, and only who, is allowed to meet or pick up your children.

Notify office and family of **travel plans**. Require that the office staff not *reveal* any travel plans or other schedules.

Be extremely careful about giving out personal information. This can be very tough on kids, as they often happily exchange information with their friends or others. Now that young people live half their lives on Internet social networks such as FaceBook and Twitter, you have to be doubly careful! You will have to be explicit on what they can say and to whom they can say it. It is very likely that you will have to control and supervise their on-line use. Remind them to be careful of strangers who want such information and to be sure to report any such queries.

Figure out with your family the best ways to **escape** from the home. Rehearse this with them. You can combine this with fire drills, something the children are already familiar with from school.

Plan how to ask for help if in public and how best to call for help if needed. **NOTE**: If your children are alone, the best stranger to ask for help is a *woman*, as women are far less likely – exponentially less likely – to be a threat. Of course, this is not the case if a woman is the threatening person or associated with that individual.

Post **emergency telephone numbers** near each extension.

Establish safe havens – places to escape to in the event of danger. If possible, enlist your neighbors in your safety plan, in watching for danger signs associated with your situation. This can include noticing strangers, observing anything unusual happening around your property, and participating as safe havens for the family if they suddenly need a place to go.

Teach your children a code word or phrase that any individual must say if they are trying to get the child to go with them. This includes neighbors and even, in some cases, relatives. For example, a person approaches your child after school and says, "Tasha, your mother and father were injured in an automobile accident. The police told me to take you to the hospital! Please come with me now." Your child should be taught to keep her distance, look for escape routes, and ask (if it was not said), "What's the word?" If the person does not immediately reply "Edsel," to make up an example, Tasha should immediately run to a safe haven and describe the person as best she can.

APPENDIX V

The Question of Positional and Compression Asphyxia
Gary M. Vilke, MD, FACEP, FAAEM

Background on Positional Asphyxia
- The concept of "Positional Asphyxia" was originally based on research that had significant methodological flaws (Reay, et al 1988)
- The premise of positional asphyxia was that if you left a patient in a hobble restraint position, he would tire, go into ventilatory failure and then asphyxiate into cardiac arrest.
- The hobble position is defined as prone with hand cuffed behind the back and ankles restrained with a device that is then pulled up and tethered to the handcuffs leaving the knees bent.
- The original research and dozens of papers since have NEVER shown hypoxia (low oxygen levels in the blood) to develop in the hobble position.
- The original research and dozens of papers since have NEVER shown hypercarbia (elevated CO_2 levels in the blood) to develop in the hobble position.
- In fact, the only paper to report that the hobble position results in positional asphyxia, actually demonstrated that oxygen saturation levels IMPROVED in all subjects who were left in a hobble position.
- Subsequent studies evaluating obese subjects also have demonstrated that when left in a hobble position, they will not asphyxiate.(Sloane, et al 2014)
- All of these studies prove that people left on their stomachs in a hobble position will not die from asphyxiation, which includes both thin and obese individuals.

Best practices
When encountered with a patient in a hobble restraint, certain assessments of a patient are critical and the documentation of the findings in the pre-hospital record is essential.
A. Assess the level of consciousness. Is the patient awake or not and is he verbal?
B. Assess perfusion. Is his skin color good and does he have a strong regular pulse?
C. Place on a monitor as soon as feasible and document first rhythm.
D. Place on pulse oximeter as soon as feasible and document O2 sat. If placing on a finger, make sure the hand is getting good perfusion through the handcuff if the O2 sat reading is low.
E. If the patient can be safely transferred to a supine position with approved 4-point restraints secured to the gurney – this is the optimal position as one has full access to the patient's airway and direct visualization of the face and access to the chest.
F. If the patient cannot be safely transferred out of the hobble position, attempt to transfer the patient in a lateral decubitus position on the gurney – preferably with the face and chest facing the EMS personnel to optimize monitoring.

G. Face down on the gurney in the hobble position is the least desirable position as the patient cannot be easily monitored or accessed if the physical status changes. If utilizing this position for transport, care must be taken to assure the airway is clear and not obstructed by sheets or the mattress. ***Despite all of the data supporting the safety of the hobble position, this is the position that will have the most scrutiny in a lawsuit if a patient deteriorates into cardiac arrest.

H. Ongoing monitoring and vigilance is important. The issue of medical concern is not the actual hobble position, as this is deemed physiologically neutral, but rather the concern is the underlying medical condition (drug induced or not) that required the patient to be hobbled in the first place.

I. These recommendations are meant to supplement, not replace, existing EMS protocols (blood glucose assessment, IV fluids, etc)

Background on Compression Asphyxia

- The concept of "Compression Asphyxia" evolved after the theory of positional asphyxia was essentially debunked. (Chan, et al. 1997, Chan et al 1998)

- The premise of compression asphyxia was that a certain amount of weight is often placed on the back of an individual to get a him into custody and handcuffed. Often this weight is multiple officers holding the person down with hands, forearms or knees. During this time period while the weight is being applied, the theory is that the subject would tire, not be able to breathe (ventilate), go into ventilatory failure and then asphyxiate into cardiac arrest.

- Research with up to 225 lbs of weight on the backs of healthy volunteers has not demonstrated physiological changes that would indicate that asphyxiation is likely with these weights. (Michalewicz, et al 2007)

- Studies with weights on the backs of normal subjects has also shown that cardiac output and blood pressure are not impacted.(Savaser, et al 2013)

- If an individual is alive, moving and breathing after the weight has been removed and then subsequently goes into cardiac arrest, the weight did not cause compressive asphyxia. ***There is not a delayed asphyxiation***, it either happens while the weight is on or it does not occur.

- Even if the weight on an individual is so great as to restrict adequate ventilation, if the subject is breathing once the weight is removed, the person will breathe out the retained CO_2 and will recover. The effects of the weight are not lasting and a breathing individual will self-correct very quickly.

- It takes a great deal of weight, consistently placed over the ventilatory muscles of the back, for a significant length of time with essentially complete impedance of ventilation without breaks to breathe in order to theoretically cause a death due to compressive asphyxia.

- If a person is vigorously and repeatedly yelling or screaming, he is moving air in and out of his lungs and thus is not meeting the "complete impedance of ventilation" criteria and thus is not in a position at that time to cause asphyxiation.

  NOTE: That being said, other medical emergencies CAN present with the *sensation* that one cannot breathe, when in fact they are ventilating fine but are suffering from a myocardial infarction or ischemia, for instance. These patients should be carefully evaluated.

Best practices

When EMS encounters a patient who had weight placed on him to get him into custody, certain assessments of a patient are critical and the documentation of the findings in the pre-hospital record is essential. Basically the patient will either be spontaneously breathing with a pulse, or not. If he is spontaneously breathing with a pulse, then he did not suffer from compression asphyxia and should be assessed and documentation should follow as per the "Best practices" for positional asphyxia (above).

If the patient is not breathing or does not have a pulse, treatment is basically standard advanced cardiac life support measures. Documentation optimally should reflect the events that led up to the cardiac arrest. Often EMS is present or staged within viewing distance of the event. If so, some of the following observations can be critically useful in evaluating the case for quality review or a subsequent legal action:

- How many officers where physically involved?
- Where were they located on the subject? (i.e. holding legs, holding head, knee on back, hands on shoulder, etc)
- How long was weight on the subject?
- Was the weight moving and shifting (did the subject arch up, roll over or was he just laying flat on his stomach)?
- At what point did the subject stop yelling in relation to the cardiac arrest?
- Was the change in status sudden or gradual over time?
- Was there weight on him at the time of the cardiac arrest and if so, how much?

Pearls

Careful monitoring – you will likely be unable to prevent a patient who is suffering from Excited Delirium Syndrome from going into cardiac arrest. Additionally, rapid recognition and treatment is unlikely to change the ultimate outcome for the patient, but careful charting and documentation is extremely beneficial for subsequent legal actions that are likely to arise.

ETCO2 - If possible, document the earliest possible end tidal CO2 level. Pre-intubation with bag-valve-mask is best if feasible, as this value if low or normal, will support that the individual did not asphyxiate, as CO2 levels are high in patients who asphyxiated.

Careful accurate documentation with details as clear as possible. These cases in which there is a cardiac arrest often end up in litigation, so clear documentation of what was observed and reported with specific details is incredibly helpful in evaluating the case.

> **Appendix V CAUTION**
>
> Medically evaluate the subject carefully, even if the person is vigorously and repeatedly yelling or screaming. It may be obvious that he is moving air in and out of his lungs and thus is not in a position at that time to cause asphyxiation – however other medical emergencies, like myocardial infarctions or ischemia can present with the sensation of difficulty breathing and should be considered during the assessment.

References

Chan TC, Vilke GM, Neuman T, Clausen JL: Restraint position and positional asphyxia. Ann Emerg Med 1997;30(5):578-586.

Chan TC, Vilke GM, Neuman T: Reexamination of custody restraint position and positional asphyxia. Am J Forensic Med Pathol 1998;19(3):201-205.

Michalewicz BA, Chan TC, Vilke GM, Levy SS, Neuman TS, Kolkhorst FW. Ventilatory and metabolic demands during aggressive physical restraint in healthy adults. J Forensic Sci 2007;52(1):171-175.

Reay DT, Howard JD, Fligner CL, Ward RJ. Effects of positional restraint on oxygen saturation and heart rate following exercise. Am J Forensic Med Pathol. 1988 Mar;9(1):16-8.

Savaser DJ, Campbell C, Castillo EM, Vilke GM, Sloane C, Neuman T, Hansen AV, Shah S, Chan TC. The effect of the prone maximal restrained position with and without weight force on cardiac output and other hemodynamic measures. J Forens Leg Med. 2013 Nov;20(8):991-5. Epub 2013 Aug 30.

Sloane C, Chan TC, Kolkhorst F, Neuman T, Castillo EM, Vilke GM. Evaluation of the Ventilatory Effects of the Prone Maximum Restraint Position (PMR) on Obese Human Subjects. Forens Sci Int 2014;237:86-9. Epub 2014;46(6):865-72. Epub 2014 Feb 14.

Endnotes

1   Schwartz, Jeffrey (with Beverly Beyette). *Brain Lock: Free Yourself from Obsessive-Compulsive Behavior*. New York: Regan Books, 1996. This is a groundbreaking book to understand this extremely troublesome problem as well as a good self-help book for your patient.

2   I have developed a method for working with individuals with borderline personality disorder, post-traumatic stress disorder, and anxiety disorder – states where the person's motto of life could be summed up in the phrase, "I can't stand right now!" Using exercises derived from Chinese physical culture (*qigong*), coupled with specific therapeutic interventions, a number of my clients have made considerable progress in developing the ability to control their emotional reactions, and even change them using voluntary control of their bodies. Contact this writer at www.edgework.info for questions on this procedure.

3   Allen, Bud, and Bosta, Diana. *Games Criminals Play: How You Can Profit by Knowing Them*. Berkeley, CA: Rae John Publishers, 1981-2002. This is one of the best books on manipulation, one where I learned a lot of the information described above.

4   Another term you may be familiar with is antisocial personality disorder. This diagnosis adequately describes the "criminal wing" of the psychopathic personality, and is a legitimate diagnosis in its own right. However, it does not adequately address the psychopath's "narcissistic wing," the qualities of callousness, sadism, grandiosity, etc., which complete the picture. In fact, some psychopaths never indulge in overtly criminal acts, at least not violent ones. They manipulate stock markets, run businesses, and become politicians instead.

5   Hare, Robert. *Without Conscience: The Disturbing World of the Psychopaths Among Us*. New York: Guilford Press, 1993. I also recommend that you visit the following page on my website. Here I have an extensive book list on a number of topics, notably many books on the subject of psychopathy and antisocial behavior. http://www.edgework.info/recommended_reading.html

6   http://www.hare.org/

7   Most stalkers are not delusional. Here are the other major categories of stalkers:

- **Relational stalkers**. Often an extension of a controlling or violent relationship, the stalker is either keeping tabs on his or her partner, or pursuing them once they have left.

- **Obsessive stalkers**. The classic stalker has a hyper-focus on the victim as prey – not necessarily to kill or even to harm, but always to control. Like others with ordinary obsessive-compulsive disorder, this stalker can be well aware that the victim does not desire contact, and may be afraid of or hate him. But just as the germ-obsessed person MUST wash his hands 50 times, despite *knowing* that they are clean, the obsessive stalker must have, must be near, or must have the attention of his victim.

- **Psychopathic stalker**. Such an individual may certainly have been in a relationship or be obsessed with his victim. But in addition, there is considerable "ego" involved – this stalker's psychological energy focuses on himself rather than the victim. A true predator, he is doing something he enjoys – because he can (for fun), or because the victim, in some way, offended him (for revenge).

8   Arieti, Silvano. *Interpretation of Schizophrenia*. 2nd ed. New York: Basic Books, Inc., 1974.

9   If you have any doubt about whether or not you should report to the police this or any other actions on the part of a patient, consult with your agency's legal advisor. If you are in private practice, the provider of your malpractice insurance almost always offers legal advice. Finally, an inexpensive solution to getting high quality legal advise is PrePaid Legal, a service that, for a minimal retainer, provides twenty-four-hour phone consultation. http://www.prepaidlegal.com

10   This elegant example is from Seattle firefighter/EMT Aaron Fields.

11   This is an actual incident. The engineer was killed trying to jump clear when the manic person wrecked the train.

12   I first heard the bubble image from the late Ron Kurtz, the originator of the Hakomi Method of Body Centered Psychotherapy, and have expanded on it to create the exercises you'll find in these pages.

13   Therapists and others working with victims of abuse or assault can use this exercise to help their patient learn to more accurately assess an internal sense of threat or trespass, something many victims of violence are unable to accurately do. See my article on this subject, "Therapeutic Self-Defense," at http://www.edgework.info/articles.html.

14   Of course, paraphrasing can be an invaluable mode of communication. This is discussed in detail in Chapter 44. However, when a patient is craving dialogue, paraphrasing will serve to alienate rather than connect with them.

15   I am aware of one case where the parasuicidal person was a physician. Law enforcement officers were able to establish that she knew <u>exactly</u> how to cut so that she did not put herself at risk. She was informed that the next "attempt" would result in prosecution. She ceased the behavior.

16   Contact the author at www.edgework.info for information regarding consultation and case planning for parasuicidal patients.

17   Lest there be any misunderstanding, this crosses all racial lines: it is a trait of "street culture," not any particular ethnicity.

18   Levinas, Emanuel. *Ethics and Infinity: Conversations with Philip Nemo*. Translated by Richard Cohen. Pgh., PA: Duquesne University Press, 1985. Grossman, David. *On Killing: The Psychological Cost of Learning to Kill in War*. Boston: Back Bay Books, 2009.

19   de Becker, Gavin. *The Gift of Fear: Survival Signals that Protect Us from Violence*. Boston, MA: Little Brown, and Company, 1997.

20   This is a very crude approximation. The definition of assault depends on the circumstances as well as the identity and abilities of you and the menacing other.

21   Edgerton, Robert B. *Sick Societies: Challenging the Myth of Primitive Harmony*. New York: The Free Press, 1992.

22   I first heard this method presented by author David Grossman. Also see his exemplary book *On Killing: The Psychological Cost of Learning to Kill in War and Society*. Santa Ana, CA: Back Bay Books, 1996.

23   I owe the image of the hands as a fence to Geoff Thompson, who has authored a number of books on his career as a doorman in violent British pubs, as well as exemplary books on self-defense.

24   I am well aware of the vehement opposition that the idea of carrying and offering cigarettes might provoke in some people (and of course, hospital policy may make this absolutely forbidden anyway). However, you may be facing a volatile, disorganized, hostile individual who is very attached to tobacco. If you are in a situation where giving a cigarette might help you or the other person avoid suffering bodily harm, is that really such a bad thing? You can – and will – answer the question yourself, but it is something to consider, at least in potentially emergent situations.

25   See the work of Dr. John Gottman of the University of Washington for a detailed discussion of contemptuous silence and stonewalling.

26   I am grateful to Dr. David Snarsch who introduced me to the concept of contact regression.

27   Weisenthal, Simon. *The Sunflower: On the Possibilities and Limits of Forgiveness*. New York: Schocken Books, 1998.

28   I am indebted to Dr. John Holttum, MD, child psychiatrist from Tacoma, Washington. I attended a presentation given by Dr. Holttum, which influenced me greatly in terms of how to "subdivide" the presenting behaviors of youth and how best to intervene with them. I must underscore that any treatment and intervention recommendations are my own, and may be at variance to those Dr. Holttum might offer.

29   For such debate:

- Louv, Richard. *Last Child in the Woods: Saving Our Children from Nature-deficit Disorder*. Chapel Hill, NC: Algonquin Books, 2005.

- Sax, Leonard. *Boys Adrift: The Five Factors Driving the Growing Epidemic of Unmotivated Boys and Underachieving Young Men*. Philadelphia: Basic Books, 2007.

30   There is increasing research and evidence that demonstrates the efficacy of a form of therapy called Eye Movement Desensitization and Reprocessing (EMDR) for working with traumatized children and adults. If you are working with traumatized individuals, juveniles or adults, referring them to therapists familiar with this method may be beneficial. http://www.emdr.com/

31   Salter, Anna. *Transforming Trauma: A Guide to Understanding and Treating Adult Survivors of Child Sexual Abuse*. Thousand Oaks, CA: Sage Publications, 1995.

32   I owe a debt for some of the basic information in this section to a form of training called PART, thanks to a workshop I attended approximately 20 years ago. I have made a number of significant changes in their basic four-part schema, as well as adding a significant amount of new data. Some of my approaches are quite different from PART, and it should not be confused with their procedures.

33   I am grateful to one of my teachers, the late Terry Dobson, who first gave me the image of violence as a locked door.

34   Amdur, Ellis and William Cooper. *Guarding the Gates: Verbal De-escalation for Security Guards*. Publication pending; see www.edgework.info for release date. This book includes the information enclosed in the present volume, tailored for security guards.

35   I am grateful to my colleague, security consultant David Rubens (http://www.meidoconsultants.com/) of London, England, for introducing me to this elegant phrase.

ABOUT THE AUTHOR

Ellis Amdur

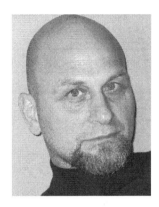

Edgework founder Ellis Amdur received his B.A. in psychology from Yale University in 1974 and his M.A. in psychology from Seattle University in 1990. He is both a National Certified Counselor and a State Certified Child Mental Health Specialist.

Since the late 1960s, Amdur has trained in various martial arts systems, spending thirteen of these years studying in Japan. He is a recognized expert in classical and modern Japanese martial traditions and has authored three iconoclastic books as well as one instructional DVD on this subject.

Since his return to America in 1988, Ellis Amdur has worked in the field of crisis intervention. He has developed a range of training and consultation services, as well as a unique style of assessment and psychotherapy. These are based on a combination of phenomenological psychology and the underlying philosophical premises of classical Japanese martial traditions. Amdur's professional philosophy can best be summed up in this idea: the development of an individual's integrity and dignity is the paramount virtue. This can only occur when people live courageously, regardless of the circumstances, and take responsibility for their roles in making the changes they desire.

Ellis Amdur is a dynamic public speaker and trainer who presents his work throughout the U.S. and internationally. He is noted for his sometimes outrageous humor as well as his profound breadth of knowledge. His vivid descriptions of aggressive and mentally ill people and his true-to-life role-playing of the behaviors in question give participants an almost firsthand experience of facing the real individuals in question.

He has written a number of works regarding de-escalation of aggression. These books are available on his website, www.edgework.info